MIX
Papier aus verantwortungsvollen Quellen
Paper from responsible sources
FSC® C105338

Dr. Vineet R.V, MDS

Assistant Professor
Department of Conservative Dentistry & Endodontics
Sree Mookambika Institute of Dental Sciences, India

Root Resorption

Pathophysiology & Management

Anchor Academic
Publishing

R.V, Vineet: Root Resorption. Pathophysiology & Management, Hamburg, Anchor
Academic Publishing 2016

Buch-ISBN: 978-3-95489-407-9
PDF-eBook-ISBN: 978-3-95489-491-8
Druck/Herstellung: Anchor Academic Publishing, Hamburg, 2016

Bibliografische Information der Deutschen Nationalbibliothek:
Die Deutsche Nationalbibliothek verzeichnet diese Publikation in der Deutschen
Nationalbibliografie; detaillierte bibliografische Daten sind im Internet über
http://dnb.d-nb.de abrufbar.

Bibliographical Information of the German National Library:
The German National Library lists this publication in the German National Bibliography.
Detailed bibliographic data can be found at: http://dnb.d-nb.de

All rights reserved. This publication may not be reproduced, stored in a retrieval system
or transmitted, in any form or by any means, electronic, mechanical, photocopying,
recording or otherwise, without the prior permission of the publishers.

Das Werk einschließlich aller seiner Teile ist urheberrechtlich geschützt. Jede Verwertung
außerhalb der Grenzen des Urheberrechtsgesetzes ist ohne Zustimmung des Verlages
unzulässig und strafbar. Dies gilt insbesondere für Vervielfältigungen, Übersetzungen,
Mikroverfilmungen und die Einspeicherung und Bearbeitung in elektronischen Systemen.

Die Wiedergabe von Gebrauchsnamen, Handelsnamen, Warenbezeichnungen usw. in
diesem Werk berechtigt auch ohne besondere Kennzeichnung nicht zu der Annahme,
dass solche Namen im Sinne der Warenzeichen- und Markenschutz-Gesetzgebung als frei
zu betrachten wären und daher von jedermann benutzt werden dürften.

Die Informationen in diesem Werk wurden mit Sorgfalt erarbeitet. Dennoch können
Fehler nicht vollständig ausgeschlossen werden und die Diplomica Verlag GmbH, die
Autoren oder Übersetzer übernehmen keine juristische Verantwortung oder irgendeine
Haftung für evtl. verbliebene fehlerhafte Angaben und deren Folgen.

Alle Rechte vorbehalten

© Anchor Academic Publishing, Imprint der Diplomica Verlag GmbH
Hermannstal 119k, 22119 Hamburg
http://www.diplomica-verlag.de, Hamburg 2016
Printed in Germany

FOREWORD

Root resorption is evolving as a troublesome dental condition because of its varied etiology and clinical presentations. However, an early diagnosis and prompt therapeutic management can provide a better prognosis. Hence, it is very essential for dental practitioners to have a thorough knowledge regarding the various factors associated with this condition so as to make a definitive diagnosis and a predictive treatment plan to curb this destructive dental condition.

This book "Root Resorption: Pathophysiology & Management" by Dr.Vineet R.V, has a compilation of evidence-based information on all facets of root resorption, that describes in depth the various types of root resorption, its etiological aspects, pathogenesis, diagnostic perspectives and a comprehensive treatment approach. Traditional principles and techniques are well reviewed as well as modern materials and methods, with a firm scientific evidence and emphasis on clinical cases. The author have maintained simplicity and readability throughout the text that would help any beginner and expert alike, in comprehending the various concepts of root resorption.

I would like to cordially congratulate Dr.Vineet R.V, for his time and effort in producing this book on such a very important subject. I wish and hope this book will be very useful for all dental practitioners.

                                      Dr. Rajesh S, MDS

                                      Professor & Head of the Department

                                      Conservative Dentistry & Endodontics

                                      Sree Mookambika Institute of Dental Sciences,

                                      Kulasekharam, Tamil Nadu, India.

FOREWORD

I have great pleasure in writing this foreword for the book " Root Resorption: Pathophysiology & Management" by Dr.Vineet R.V. This book gives the basic concepts as well as latest research finding on the etiology, pathogenesis and management of various forms of root resorption. This book is a valuable source of reference for all dental professionals, who mostly encounters the diagnostic dilemma of root resorption.The author has taken tremendous effort in preparing this book, focusing attention on evaluation of various intricate concepts of root resorption as well as thoughtfully dividing them into logical sequences so that all readers can comprehend the various aspects regardless of their personal level of knowledge. I would like to appreciate Dr.Vineet R.V, for his general and in-depth knowledge and experience as well as on this well-conceived and scientifically written book. I wish and hope this book finds the deserved use and popularity.

Dr. Elizabeth Koshy, MDS

Principal/ Dean

Sree Mookambika Institute of Dental Sciences,

Kulasekharam, Tamil Nadu, India.

CONTENTS

ACKNOWLEDGEMENTS 7

PROLOGUE 8

CHAPTER 1: WHAT IS ROOT RESORPTION? 9

CHAPTER 2: PATHOGENESIS OF ROOT RESORPTION 10
    THEORIES FOR THE RESISTANCE OF THE ROOT TO RESORPTION 10
    CELLS INVOLVED IN ROOT RESORPTION 11
    REGULATION OF OSTEOCLAST AND ODONTOCLAST ACTIVITY 12
    MECHANISM OF ROOT RESORPTION 15
    FACTORS REGULATING ROOT RESORPTION 16
    REQUIREMENTS FOR THE PRESENCE OF ROOT RESORPTION 19

CHAPTER 3: CLASSIFICATION OF ROOT RESORPTION 22

CHAPTER 4: INTERNAL ROOT RESORPTION 28
    ETIOLOGY AND PATHOGENESIS 29
    HISTOLOGIC MANIFESTATIONS 31
    INTERNAL INFLAMMATORY RESORPTION 32
    INTERNAL REPLACEMENT RESORPTION 33
    HYPOTHESES REGARDING ORIGIN OF METAPLASTIC HARD TISSUES 35
    CLINICAL FEATURES OF INTERNAL RESORPTION 36
    RADIOGRAPHIC FEATURES OF INTERNAL RESORPTION 37
    TREATMENT PERSPECTIVES 40
    INSTRUMENTATION OF TEETH WITH INTERNAL RESORPTION 40
    INTRACANAL MEDICAMENTS FOR INTERNAL RESORPTION 41
    PERMANENT FILLING OF ROOT CANAL AND INTERNAL RESORPTION 42
    TREATMENT 43

CHAPTER 5: EXTERNAL ROOT RESORPTION 46
    DIFFERENCE BETWEEN INTERNAL AND EXTERNAL ROOT RESORPTION 46
    EXTERNAL SURFACE RESORPTION 46
    EXTERNAL CERVICAL RESORPTION 48
    EXTERNAL INFLAMMATORY RESORPTION 55
    EXTERNAL REPLACEMENT RESORPTION 61

CHAPTER 6: CLINICAL VARIANTS OF ROOT RESORPTION 62
    PULPAL INFECTION ROOT RESORPTION 62
    PERIODONTAL INFECTION ROOT RESORPTION 64
    ORTHODONTIC PRESSURE ROOT RESORPTION... 65
    IMPACTED TOOTH OR TUMOR PRESSURE ROOT RESORPTION.......................... 66
    ANKYLOTIC ROOT RESORPTION 67

CHAPTER 7: TRANSIENT APICAL BREAKDOWN 69

CHAPTER 8: RESORPTION DUE TO SYSTEMIC CAUSES 70

CHAPTER 9: IDIOPATHIC ROOT RESORPTION 71

CONCLUSION 72

REFERENCES... 73

ABOUT THE AUTHOR 78

ACKNOWLEDGEMENTS

"Gratitude is the memory of the heart."
Jean Baptiste Massieu

I take this moment to thank personally each and everyone who had helped me during the various stages of this work. I sincerely thank my postgraduate guide Dr. Moksha Nayak. Her tireless pursuit for perfection, professional insight and immense support were a source of constant inspiration to me. Her insistence on learning the basics, thinking logically and working systematically has always spurred me reach the highest level of excellence. It is my privilege and honor to express my gratitude to Dr. Krishnaprasad L, for his encouragement, support and timely help, whenever needed.

I am deeply indebted to my beloved parents and my sister who have forever stood by me in my times of despair and no amount of words will suffice the gratitude that I have towards them for their love and never ending support. I will always remain grateful to my entire family for their support and significant contribution in making me reach this level in my life.

Above all I would like to thank almighty who always held in reserve blessings for me and gave me the strength and direction all the years of my life.

PROLOGUE

Root resorption is a perplexing problem for all dental practitioners. It is the loss of dental hard tissues as a result of clastic activities. It might occur as a physiologic or pathologic phenomenon.[1] Root resorption in the primary dentition is a normal physiologic process. The initiating factors involved in physiologic root resorption in the primary dentition are not completely understood, although the process appears to be regulated by cytokines and transcription factors that are similar to those involved in bone remodeling.[2,3] Unlike bone that undergoes continuous physiologic remodeling throughout life, root resorption of permanent teeth does not occur naturally and is invariably inflammatory in nature. Thus, root resorption in the permanent dentition is a pathologic event; if untreated, this might result in the premature loss of the affected teeth.[4] This is a very frustrating condition to both dentist and patient. In many cases the dentist has limited treatment options to offer and the patient experiences a condition that is not the result of their actions or neglect. Although this pathologic condition has been reported for more than a century, our knowledge on the pathogenesis of this disease is, unfortunately, surprisingly thin.[5]

CHAPTER 1: WHAT IS ROOT RESORPTION?

A condition associated with either a physiologic or a pathologic process that results in loss of substance from a tissue such as dentine, cementum or alveolar bone.[6] (Trope & Chivian 1984)

Root resorption is defined as a condition of dental complication associated with either a physiological or pathological activity of the tooth resorbing cells, which results in loss of cementum and /or dentine.[7] (L.Tronstad 1988)

Root resorption is a physiologic or pathologic process that results in a loss of substance from dentine or cementum.[8] (P.Rygh 1997)

The process of removal of cementum and/or dentin through physiological or pathological activity of tooth resorbing cells, which may be called dentinoclasts.[9] (Laux et al 2000)

The destruction of the cementum or dentin by cementoclastic or osteoclastic activity. It may result in a shortening or blunting of the root. Lateral root resorption may also occur, resulting in a loss of root substance along the side or length of the root. (Mosby's Medical Dictionary, 8th ed.)

It is the process of dissolution of the root of a tooth; either external, with loss or blunting of the apical portion, or internal, with loss of dentin from the inside (pulpal) part of the root area. (Stedman's medical dictionary, 2006)

Root resorption is the loss of hard dental tissue (ie, cementum and dentin) as a result of odontoclastic action.[10] (Pitt Ford 2007)

CHAPTER 2: PATHOGENESIS OF ROOT RESORPTION

The etiology as well as the pathophysiology of root resorption is multifactorial. A comprehensive knowledge of the pathogenesis of root resorption requires the understanding of the following concepts.

THEORIES FOR THE RESISTANCE OF THE ROOT TO RESORPTION

The three hard tissues involved in resorption

- ❖ Bone
- ❖ Cementum
- ❖ Dentin

Unlike deciduous teeth, permanent teeth rarely undergo root resorption . Even in the presence of periradicular inflammation, resorption will occur primarily on the bone side of the attachment apparatus and the root will be resistant to it.

▶ *First hypothesis* is that remnants of the epithelial root sheath surround the root like a net, therefore imparting a resistance to resorption and subsequent ankylosis[11]

▶ *Second hypothesis by Andreason*[12]
This theory is based on the premise that the precementum and predentin are essential elements in the resistance of the root to resorption. It has long been noted that osteoclasts will not adhere to or resorb unmineralized matrix. Since the most external aspect of cementum is covered by a layer of cementoblasts over a zone of non-mineralized cementoid, a surface that provides satisfactory conditions for osteoclast binding is not present. Internally, the dentin is covered by predentin matrix, which possesses a similar organic surface. Even in the presence of inflammation, an intact root is resistant to resorption. Another function of the cemental layer is related to its ability to inhibit the movement of toxins if present in the root canal space into the surrounding periodontal tissues.

CELLS INVOLVED IN ROOT RESORPTION

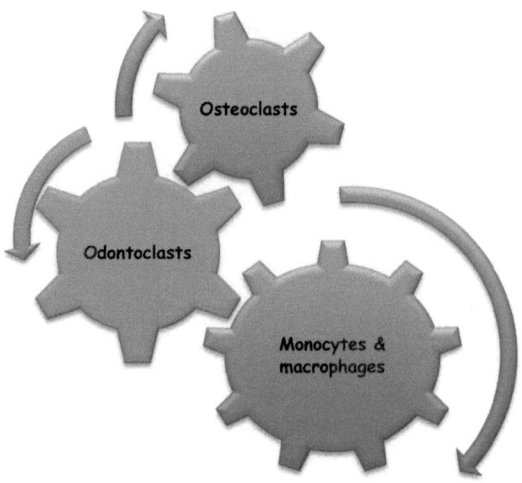

Osteoclasts are multinuclear cells responsible for resorption of bone, while odontoclasts are corresponding cells resorbing dental hard tissues. The multinuclear cells are formed by fusion of mononuclear cells. Microscopic studies of odontoclasts using three-dimensional reconstruction have shown that several mononuclear odontoclast precursor cells may undergo fusion simultaneously with each other and with multinuclear cells. Mononuclear odontoclasts can also actively resorb dental hard tissue, although during progressive resorption most cells have several nuclei. Domon et al. showed that in deciduous teeth undergoing resorption, the mean number of nuclei per odontoclast was 5.3, and only 2.9% of the resorbing cells were mononuclear.[6] Comparative studies on cell ultrastructure have shown that odontoclasts resorbing dentin or cementum are similar to those resorbing enamel. Close similarity to bone osteoclasts was also documented.

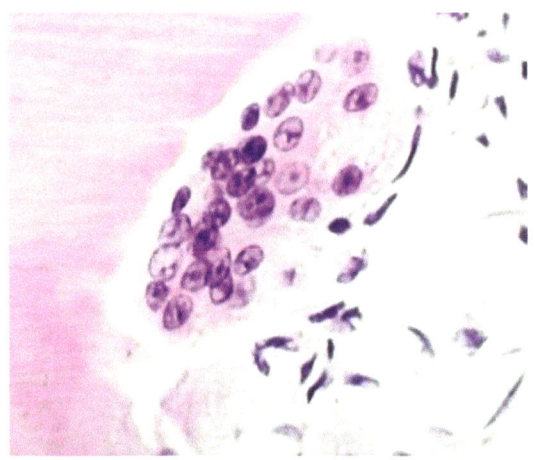

(Courtesy of Dr.P L Lukinmaa)

A study of key enzymes in the resorptive process,acid phosphatase, cathepsin K, and matrix metalloproteinase-9 in osteoclasts and odontoclasts during physiological root resorption in human deciduous teeth found that there were no differences in the expression of these molecules between the two cells. Based on available knowledge about osteoclasts and odontoclasts, there does not seem to be any difference between these cells other than their site of action in the body; they share a common mechanism in cellular resorption of bone and teeth.[7]

REGULATION OF OSTEOCLAST AND ODONTOCLAST ACTIVITY

Osteoclasts do not have a receptor for direct binding of PTH (Parathyroid hormone), therefore the stimulation of osteoclasts by PTH is indirect. PTH or PTHrP bind to osteoblasts; bone forming cells, which increases their expression of 'Receptor Activator of Nuclear Factor k B Ligand,'(RANKL), which can bind to the RANK receptor of osteoclast precursor cells, the latter become active osteoclasts through cell fusion.[8]

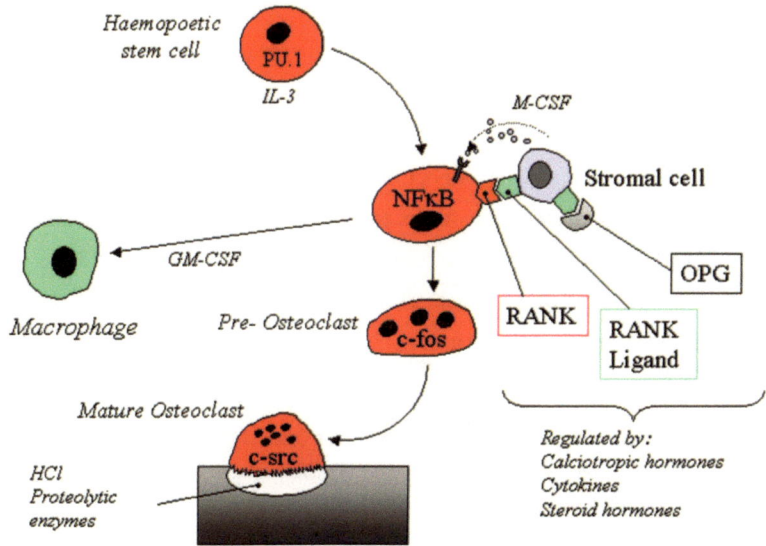

(Courtesy Teitelbaum science)

Osteoprotegerin (OPG) is a glycoprotein that is a secreted member of the tumor necrosis factor (TNF) receptor superfamily and has a variety of biological functions including the regulation of bone turnover. OPG is a potent inhibitor of osteoclastic bone resorption by competitively inhibiting the association of the OPG ligand with the RANK receptor on osteoclasts and osteoclast precursors. Fukushima et al. reported that periodontal ligament cells express RANKL during physiological root resorption of primary teeth but decrease OPG expression.[9]

It has recently been shown that TNF-α contributes to the development of osteoclasts and multinuclear cells with dentin resorbing capacity. Komine et al. demonstrated that human TNF-α markedly stimulated the formation of mononuclear preosteoclast-like cells (POC) in the presence of conditioned medium of osteoblastic cells. TNF-α also aided differentiation of hematopoietic progenitor cells into POCs. The POC induced by human TNF-α formed multinuclear cells, which showed dentine-resorbing activity after co-culture with primary osteoblasts. Extremely low levels of TNF-α increased the level of mRNA for calcitonin receptor and cathepsin-K of the POC. The effects of both RANKL and TNF-α on osteoclast development are inhibited by OPG.[10]

Studies on the role of macrophage colony stimulating factor (M-CSF) in osteoclast activation have been to some extent contradictory. It has been postulated by Udagawa et al that M-CSF is not involved in the activation of osteoclasts by osteoblasts.[11] However, studies by Tsurukai et al showed that M-CSF and soluble RANKL produced by osteoblasts were essential for osteoclast precursor cell formation and for osteoclast formation. Interestingly, fibroblast growth factor 2 (FGF-2) has been shown to have a dualistic effect on osteoclast differentiation and activation. In the co-culture system of osteoblasts and bone marrow cells, FGF-2 stimulated osteoclast formation from the latter.[12]

The effect of FGF-2 on osteoclast formation is inhibited by OPG and by cyclo-oxygenase 2 (COX-2) inhibitor, which indicates that FGF-2 stimulates osteoclasts partially by prostaglandin production. However, FGF-2 also exhibits a direct inhibitory action on osteoclast precursors by counteracting M-CSF signaling.

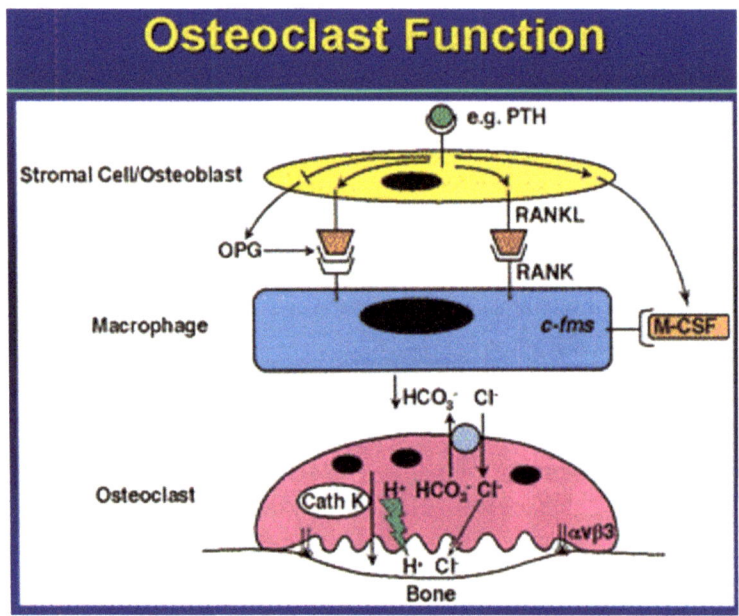

(courtesy Teitelbaum science)

Prostaglandin E2 upregulates the production of RANKL messenger RNA in osteoblasts, thereby stimulating osteoclast activation. A number of other substances have also been shown to regulate osteoclast activity. Activators and stimulators of multinuclear resorbing cells include PTH, PTHrP, interleukin (IL)-1, IL-6 and IL-11, platelet-derived growth factor (PDGF), 1,25 hydroxy vitamin D3, glucocorticoids and substance P (31–43). While calcitonin, estrogen, interferon, IL-4, IL-8, IL-10, IL-18 and corticosteroids are involved in the inhibition of osteoclast/odontoclast cells.[13]

Inflammation caused by a microbial infection is regarded as a major factor in several types of progressive resorptions. Increased RANKL production and stimulation of osteoclastogenesis have been demonstrated by incubating PDL cells with whole cells of Prevotella intermedia or lipopolysaccharide from P. nigrescens. Increased RANKL production has also been shown with stimulation by a Gram positive bacterial species, Streptococcus pyogenes. Interestingly, it was recently shown that surface associated (capsular) material from Staphylococcus aureus, another Gram-positive species, stimulates osteoclast differentiation by a RANKL-independent mechanism.[14] Nair et al. reported that cell surface-associated proteins (SAP) from S. aureus are potent stimulators of bone resorption.[15]

MECHANISM OF ROOT RESORPTION

The root resorption process generally has two stages:[19]

▶ Degradation of the inorganic structure - Hydroxyapatite

▶ Degradation of the organic structure - Type I collagen

Degradation of the inorganic structure:

By producing an acidic microenvironment

▶ Highly active polarized proton pump

☐ Within the ruffled border

▶ Carbonic anhydrase II

☐ Present intracellular

☐ Catalyses $CO_2 \longrightarrow H_2CO_3$

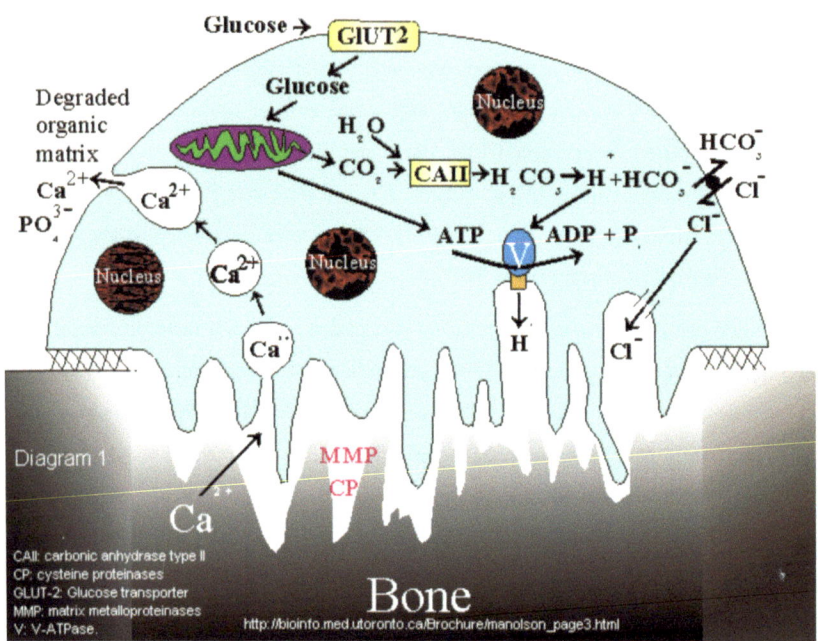

Diagram 1

CAII: carbonic anhydrase type II
CP: cysteine proteinases
GLUT-2: Glucose transporter
MMP: matrix metalloproteinases
V: V-ATPase.

Degradation of the organic structure:

By three groups of proteinase enzymes

► Act at / just below neutral pH

☐ Collagenase

☐ Matrix metalloproteinase (MMP)

► Act at acidic pH

☐ Cysteine proteinase

FACTORS REGULATING ROOT RESORPTION

Systemic regulatory factors:

► Promote resorption

☐ Parathyroid hormone (PTH)

☐ 1,25-dihydroxyvitamin D3

► Inhibit resorption

☐ Calcitonin

Parathyroid hormone (PTH):

► Stimulates osteoblasts via receptor –mediated, cAMP-dependent pathway which causes:

☐ Increase of neutral proteases

☐ Decrease protease inhibitor and matrix deposition

► Acts on osteoclasts and increases carbonic anhydrase II activity

► Promotes fusion of marrow cells and forms osteoclastic multinucleated giant cells

1,25-dihydroxyvitamin D3: Increases resorptive activity of osteoclasts already present

Calcitonin: Inhibits cytoplasmic motility and produces cell retraction

Local regulatory factors:

► Cytokines

☐ Macrophage colony-stimulating factor (M-CSF)

☐ Interleukin 6 (IL-6)

☐ Interleukin 1 (IL-1)

☐ TNF –α

► Arachidonic acid metabolites (PGE2)

► Endotoxin (lipopolysaccharides)

Cytokines

► Macrophage colony-stimulating factor (M-CSF)

☐ Proliferation of osteoclast progenitor

☐ Subsequent differentiation into mature osteoclasts

▶ Interleukin 6 (IL-6)

☐ Acts on osteoblastic stromal cells to induce osteoclast differentiation factor

☐ Indirectly helps in the differentiation of oseoclast

▶ Interleukin 1 (IL-1)

☐ Acts indirectly through the osteoblast

☐ Act directly on the osteoclast

☐ Stimulates the production and release of prostaglandin E2 (PG2)

▶ TNF –α

☐ Stimulate osteoclastic activity

Prostaglandins

▶ PGE2

☐ Stimulates formation of osteoclasts

Enhancing the fusion of osteoclastic precursors

☐ Increases the resorbing activity of existing cells

Bacterial endotoxin / LPS (lipopolysaccharide)

☐ Induction of osteolytic factors

▶ Lysosomal enzyme release

▶ Collagenase release from macrophages

▶ Osteoblastic secretion of osteolytic factors

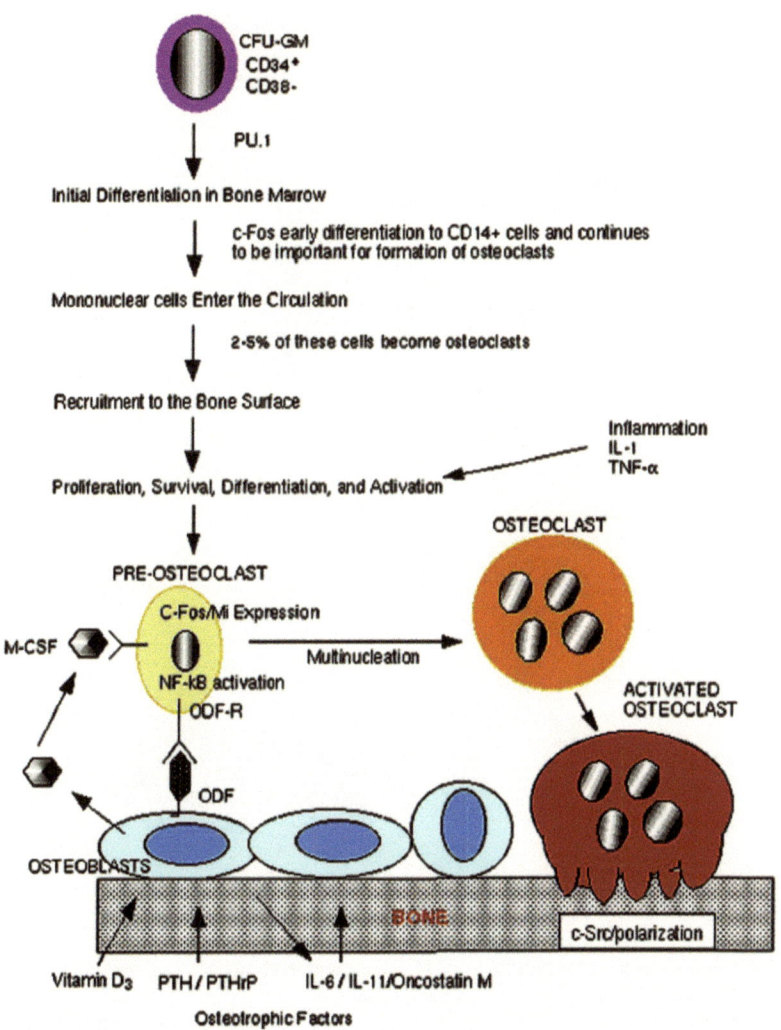

(courtesy Shafers oral pathology)

REQUIREMENTS FOR THE PRESENCE OF ROOT RESORPTION

▶ The loss or alteration of the protective layer

☐ pre-cementum

☐ pre-dentin

▶ Sustained inflammation must occur to the unprotected root surface

Loss or alteration of the protective layer (precementum or predentin)

▶ Directly

☐ due to the trauma of a dental injury

☐ Especially intrusive injury

▶ Indirectly

☐ Inflammation in reaction to the traumatic injury

▶ varies according to the stimulus it is exposed to after the injury

▶ has the potential to cause extensive damage to the protective layer

Inflammatory response

The inflammatory response caused by the dental injury can be divided into two critical phases

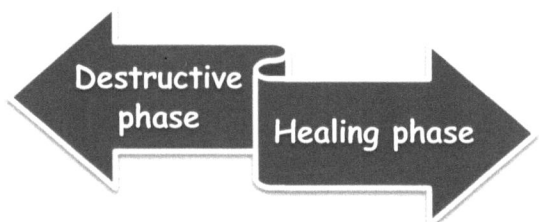

Destructive phase:

▶ where active resorption between the dried-out cells with multinucleated giant cells takes place

▶ This destruction will continue as long as there is stimulus present to allow the inflammation to develop

▶ stimulus only exist for a short period of time

☐ Healing will take place without intervention by the dentist

▶ If the inflammatory stimulus is long-standing

☐ the destructive root resorption will continue until either no root structure remains or the stimulus is removed by the intervention of the dentist.

Healing phase:

The critical factor in determining the outcome after a dental traumatic injury has occurred is the type of cells that repopulate the root surface during the healing phase

Cementoblasts

The type of healing is termed

☐ cemental healing or surface resorption will occur

☐ the outcome will be favorable

Osteoblasts

▶ the conditions for healing will be unfavorable

▶ Ankylosis, replacement **resorption** or osseous replacement will occur

The type of tissue that will cover the root surface is dependent on

☐ the surface area of the root damage

▶ destruction of over 20% of the root surface is required for osseous replacement to occur

☐ the relative proximity of the cells to the root; i.e. how far and how fast the cells can travel in order to cover the damaged root surface

Surface area of root damage is dependent on:

☐ the scale of the initial injury which cannot be reversed.

☐ the extent of the destructive inflammatory response.

The way in which the tooth is handled is of crucial importance. There is opportunity for the initial inflammation to be minimized by actions taken immediately after the injury by the pharmacological manipulation of the inflammatory response.

CHAPTER 3: CLASSIFICATION OF ROOT RESORPTION

I. **Based on the anatomical region of occurrence**

- Internal root resorption
- External root resorption
  - Cervical root resorption
  - External apical root resorption

II. **According to Kronfeld: site of origin**

- External root resorption
  - Transient
  - Progressive
- Internal root resorption
  - Metaplastic
  - Internal replacement
  - Internal inflammatory
- Resorption due to trauma

III. **Classification based on etiology (Trope & Chivian 1994)**

- Local causes of root resorption
- Orthodontic tooth movement
- Impacted tooth
- Tumours or cysts
- Inflammation
- External
  - Apical
  - Lateral
  - Cervical
- Internal
  - Dentoalveolar ankylosis
  - Replacement resorption
- Systemic causes of root resorption
- Idiopathic resorption

IV. Classification by Ne et al, 1999

- ❖ Internal resorption
    - ➢ Root canal (internal) replacement resorption
    - ➢ Internal inflammatory resorption
- ❖ External resorption (according to its clinical and histologic manifestations)
    - ➢ External surface resorption
    - ➢ External inflammatory root resorption
- ❖ cervical resorption with or without a vital pulp
    - ➢ invasive cervical root resorption
- ❖ External apical root resorption (EARR)
    - ➢ Replacement resorption
    - ➢ Ankylosis
- ❖ Transient apical breakdown (TAB)
- ❖ Combined internal and external resorption

V. Based on stimulating factors (Fuss et al 2003)

- ❖ Pulpal infection root resorption
- ❖ Periodontal infection root resorption
- ❖ Orthodontic pressure root resorption
- ❖ Impacted tooth/tumor pressure root resorption
- ❖ Ankylotic root resorption

VI. According to Cohen

- ❖ Internal
- ❖ External
    - ➢ Surface
    - ➢ Inflammatory
    - ➢ Replacement
        - ▪ transient
        - ▪ progressive
- ❖ Invasive
- ❖ Idiopathic
- ❖ Pressure

VII. According to Andreason & Andreason (1992)

- ❖ Non-invasive
  - ➢ Surface resorption
- ❖ Invasive
  - ➢ Replacement resorption
  - ➢ Inflammatory resorption

VIII. Classification by Pohl et al (2005)

- ❖ Replacement resorption / ankylosis
- ❖ Infection related resorption
  - ➢ Early infection related resorption
  - ➢ Tunneling infection related resorption
  - ➢ Complete replacement resorption succeeded by cervical resorption

IX. Frank's classification of extra-canal invasive root resorption

- ❖ Supraosseous
- ❖ Intraosseous
- ❖ Crestal

X. Heithersay classification for external cervical resorption

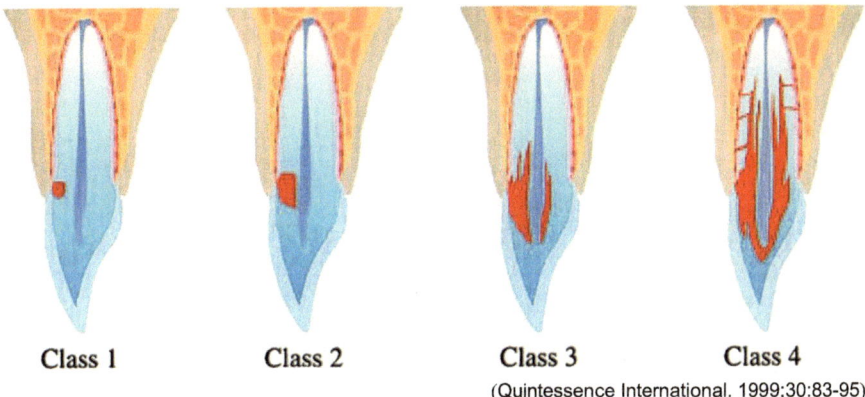

(Quintessence International. 1999;30:83-95)

Class 1: Localized defect entirely within the coronal third of the tooth

Class 2: Localized defect close to the cervical margin

Class 3: Localized, medium-sized defect located in the coronal and mid-root dentin with a small subepithelial opening on the root.

Class 4: Large defect extending apically.

XI. According to Castelluci

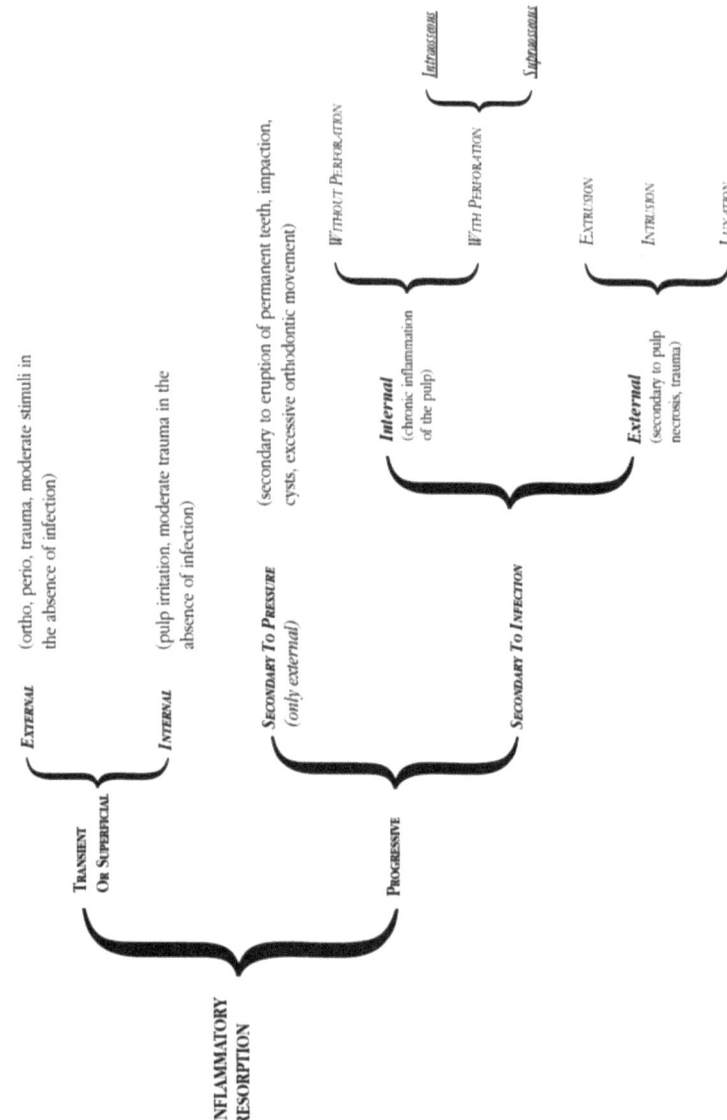

RESORPTION WITH ANKYLOSIS AND REPLACEMENT (secondary to extensive necrosis of the periodontal ligament, subluxation, or avulsion)

EXTRACANAL INVASIVE RESORPTION, CERVICAL RESORPTION (TRONSTAD), OR EXTERNAL-INTERNAL RESORPTION (FRANK)

{ **SUPRAOSSEOUS OR CRESTAL**

INTRAOSSEOUS }
{ *TRAUMA*
PERIODONTAL INFECTION
ORTHODONTICS
BLEACHING
IDIOPATHIC }

CHAPTER 4: INTERNAL ROOT RESORPTION

Internal root resorption is the progressive destruction of intraradicular dentin and dentinal tubules along the middle and apical thirds of the canal walls as a result of clastic activities. Internal root resorption has been described as intraradicular or apical according to the location in which the condition is observed. Intraradicular internal resorption is an inflammatory condition that results in progressive destruction of intraradicular dentin and dentinal tubules along the middle and apical thirds of the canal walls.The resorptive spaces might be filled by granulation tissue only or in combination with bone-like or cementum-like mineralized tissues. The condition is more frequently observed in male than female subjects.[22] Although intraradicular internal root resorption is a relatively rare clinical entity even after traumatic injury, a higher prevalence of the condition has been associated with teeth that had undergone specific treatment procedures such as autotransplantation.[23]

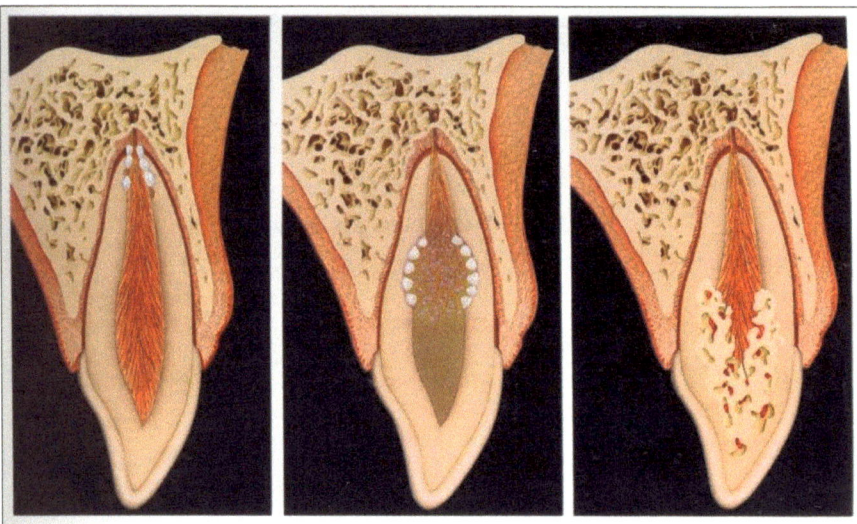

Three types of root canal (internal) resorption may develop subsequent to trauma: internal surface resorption, internal inflammatory resorption, and internal ankylosis.

(Courtesy Dr.Zvi Fuss)

Cabrini et al. amputated the coronal pulps of 28 teeth and dressed the radicular pulp stumps with calcium hydroxide mixed with distilled water. Eight of the 28 teeth extracted between 49 and 320 days after the procedure demonstrated histologic evidence of internal resorption.[26] Calixskan and Turkuin examined the prognosis of endodontic treatment on 25 teeth with nonperforating and perforating internal resorption. They reported that the most commonly affected teeth were maxillary incisors.[27] The small sample sizes in these studies precluded definitive conclusions to be drawn on the prevalence of internal root resorption. Moreover, diagnosis of internal resorption in most of the earlier studies was based solely on 2-dimensional radiographic evidence, without complementary 3-dimensional radiographic and/or histologic support.[17] Further epidemiologic studies are required to identify whether there are racial predilections in the manifestation of intraradicular internal resorption.

Compared with intraradicular internal resorption, apical internal resorption is a fairly common occurrence in teeth with periapical lesions. The authors examined the extent of internal resorption in 75 roots (69 roots with radiolucent periapical lesions and 6 vital control roots) and graded the severity of resorption on a 4-point scale. They concluded that 75% of teeth associated with periapical lesions had internal apical resorption and that vital teeth had statistically less apical internal resorption than teeth with periapical lesions. Severe internal resorption could be identified in 48% of those cases with periapical lesions. Conversely, only 1 root in the control group displayed mild internal resorption, which was speculated to be transient in nature as a result of trauma.[18]

ETIOLOGY AND PATHOGENESIS

For internal root resorption to occur, the outermost protective odontoblast layer and the predentin of the canal wall must be damaged, resulting in exposure of the underlying mineralized dentin to odontoclasts. The precise injurious events necessary to bring about such damages have not been completely elucidated. Various etiologic factors have been proposed for the loss of predentin, including trauma, caries and periodontal infections, excessive heat generated during restorative procedures on vital teeth, calcium hydroxide procedures, vital root resections, anachoresis, orthodontic treatment, cracked teeth, or simply idiopathic dystrophic changes within normal pulps. In a study of 25 teeth with internal resorption, trauma was found to be the most common predisposing factor that was responsible for 45% of the cases examined.[19] The suggested etiologies in the other cases were inflammation as a result of carious lesions (25%) and periodontal lesions (14%). The cause of the internal resorption in the remaining teeth was unknown. Other reports in the literature also support the view that trauma and pulpal inflammation/infection are the major contributory factors in the initiation of internal resorption.[20]

Wedenberg and Lindskog reported that internal root resorption could be a transient or a progressive event.[21] In an in vivo primate study, the root canals were accessed in 32 incisors with the predentin intentionally damaged. The access cavities in half of the teeth were sealed; the other half were left open to the oral cavity. The teeth were extracted at intervals of 1, 2, 6, and 10 weeks. The authors noted only a transient colonization of the damaged dentin by multinucleated clastic cells in the teeth that had been sealed (ie, transient internal root resorption). Those teeth were free from bacterial contamination, and no signs of active hard tissue resorption occurred. In the teeth that were left unsealed during the experimental period, there were signs of extensive bacterial contamination of pulpal tissue and dentinal tubules. Those teeth demonstrated extensive and prolonged colonization of the damaged dentin surface by clastic cells and signs of mineralized tissue resorption (progressive internal root resorption). Damage to the odontoblast layer and predentin of the canal wall is a prerequisite for the initiation of internal root resorption. However, the advancement of internal root resorption depends on bacterial stimulation of the clastic cells involved in hard tissue resorption. Without this stimulation, the resorption will be self-limiting.[22]

For internal resorption to occur, the pulp tissue apical to the resorptive lesion must have a viable blood supply to provide clastic cells and their nutrients, whereas the infected necrotic coronal pulp tissue provides stimulation for those clastic cells. Bacteria might enter the pulp canal through dentinal tubules, carious cavities, cracks, fractures, and lateral canals. In the absence of a bacterial stimulus, the resorption will be transient and might not advance to the stage that can be diagnosed clinically and radiographically. Therefore, the pulp apical to the site of resorption must be vital for the resorptive lesion to progress. If left untreated, internal resorption might continue until the inflamed connective tissue filling the resorptive defect degenerates, advancing the lesion in an apical direction. Ultimately, if left untreated, the pulp tissue apical to the resorptive lesion will undergo necrosis, and the bacteria will infect the entire root canal system, resulting in apical periodontitis.[23]

HISTOLOGIC MANIFESTATIONS

Wedenberg and Zetterqvist studied, internal root resorption lesions in both primary and permanent teeth using light microscopy, scanning electron microscopy, and enzyme histochemistry. The study examined 6 primary and 7 permanent teeth that were extracted as a result of progressive internal resorption. The histologic appearance and histochemical profiles of the primary and permanent teeth were identical, but the resorption process generally occurred at a faster rate in the primary teeth.[12] Pulpal tissues in all the teeth were inflamed to varying degrees, with the inflammatory infiltrate consisting predominantly of lymphocytes and macrophages, with some neutrophils. The inflammation was associated with dilated blood vessels, and in 11 of the cases, bacteria were evident either in the necrotic coronal pulp tissue or within the dentinal tubules adjacent to the lesion. The granulation tissue in the pulp cavities contained fewer blood vessels than in normal pulp tissue and resembled periodontal connective tissues, with comparatively more cells and fibers. Indeed, the periodontal membrane was continuous with the tissue in the pulp cavities in all but 2 teeth through either the apical foramen or perforations of the external root surfaces as a result of the resorption process.[24]

A distinguishing feature of all the lesions examined was the presence of numerous, large, multinucleated odontoclasts occupying resorption lacunae on the canal walls. The odontoclasts displayed evidence of active resorption and were accompanied by mononuclear inflammatory cells in the adjacent connective tissue. Both types of cell displayed tartrate-resistant acid phosphatase activity. There were no predentin or odontoblasts on the dentinal walls. Of interest was the presence of a metaplastic mineralized tissue that resembled bone or cementum. The metaplastic mineralized tissues incompletely lined the pulp cavity in all cases, and islands of calcified tissues were identified from the pulp in 3 teeth. Similar metaplastic mineralized tissues were reported by Cvek et al, with "ankylosis of the canal walls" similar to what was observed along the external root surfaces. On the basis of those results, 2 types of internal root resorption were described by Ne et al and Heithersay, internal (root canal) inflammatory resorption and internal (root canal) replacement resorption.[28]

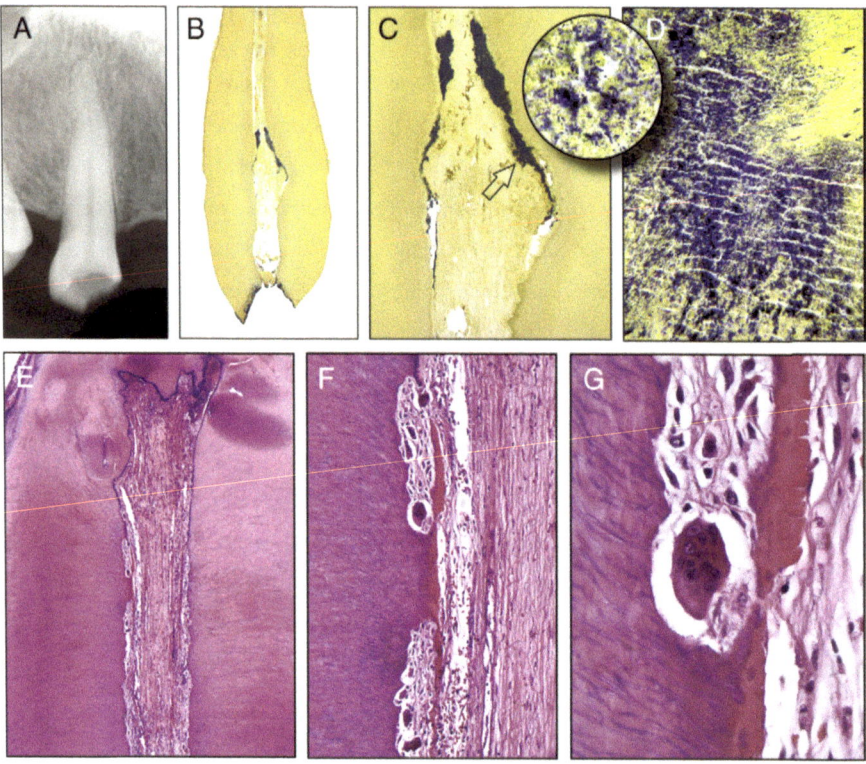

Light microscopy images of a case with internal inflammatory resorption. (a) Maxillary canine with caries penetrating the pulp. (b) Sections were taken along the buccolingual plane. (c) Coronal third of the root. Dense bacterial biofilm was present on the canal walls. (d) High magnification of the area indicated by the arrow . (e) Apical third of the root. (f) Magnification of the left root canal wall. The odontoblast layer was absent, with only some remaining predentin.Resorption lacunae can be observed along the canal wall. (g) Higher magnification of the upper lacuna in. Large multinucleated resorbing cell (odontoclast) and granulation tissue consisting of fibroblasts and chronic inflammatory cells can be seen.(courtesy *Internal Root Resorption: A Review by* Dr.Shanon Patel)

INTERNAL INFLAMMATORY RESORPTION

This type of resorption is characterized by the radiographic appearance of an ovalshaped enlargement within the pulp chamber. The condition might go unnoticed until the lesion has advanced significantly, resulting in a perforation or symptoms of acute or chronic apical periodontitis after the entire pulp has undergone necrosis and the pulp space has become infected. If resorption occurs in the coronal portion of the tooth, the latter might exhibit a pinkish hue that is classically described as the pink tooth of Mummery after the 19th century anatomist James Howard Mummery, who first reported the phenomenon.[29] Internal root canal inflammatory resorption involves a progressive loss of intraradicular dentin without adjunctive deposition of hard tissues adjacent to the resorptive sites. It is frequently associated with chronic pulpal inflammation, and bacteria might be identified from the granulation tissues when the lesion is progressive to the extent that it is identifiable with routine radiographs. Although chronic inflammation is commonly present in pulpal infections, it alone does not provide the conditions necessary for mediating root canal inflammatory resorption. Other conditions must be present simultaneously to initiate the event.[30] This probably explains why root canal inflammatory resorption is less frequently observed than external inflammatory root resorption (EIRR). The coronal part of the pulp is usually necrotic, whereas the apical part of the pulp must remain vital for the resorptive lesion to progress and enlarge. One hypothesis suggests that the necrotic coronal part of the infected pulp provides a stimulus for inflammation in the apical part of the pulp. An alternative hypothesis is based on the recent understanding that osteocytes participate in bone homeostasis by inhibiting osteoclastogenesis. In the presence of living osteocytes, osteoclasts fail to produce actin rings, which are the hallmark of active resorbing cells.[31]

Conversely, apoptosis of osteocytes induces the secretion of osteoclastogenic cytokines that trigger bone resorption. Similar to osteocytes, dental pulp cells and odontoblasts undergo apoptosis during tooth development as well as in response to certain types of injury. Thus, it is possible that odontoblasts or pulpal fibroblasts undergoing apoptosis as a result of trauma or caries produce cytokines that initiate an internal resorptive response in the apical part of the pulp. Internal resorption only occurs when the predentin adjacent to the site of chronic inflammation is lost as a result of traucma or other unknown etiologic factors.[32]

INTERNAL REPLACEMENT RESORPTION

Internal root canal replacement resorption is characterized by an irregular radiographic enlargement of the pulp chamber, with discontinuity of the normal canal space. Because the resorption process is initiated within the root canal, the defect includes part of the canal space, and hence the outline of the original canal appears distorted. The enlarged canal space appeared radiographically to be obliterated by a fuzzy-appearing material of mild to moderate radiodensity. This form of resorption is typically asymptomatic, and the affected teeth might respond normally to thermal and/or electric pulp testing unless the resorptive process results in crown or root perforation.[33]

Root canal replacement resorption appears to be caused by a low-grade inflammation of the pulpal tissues such as chronic irreversible pulpitis or partial necrosis.

Histologic features

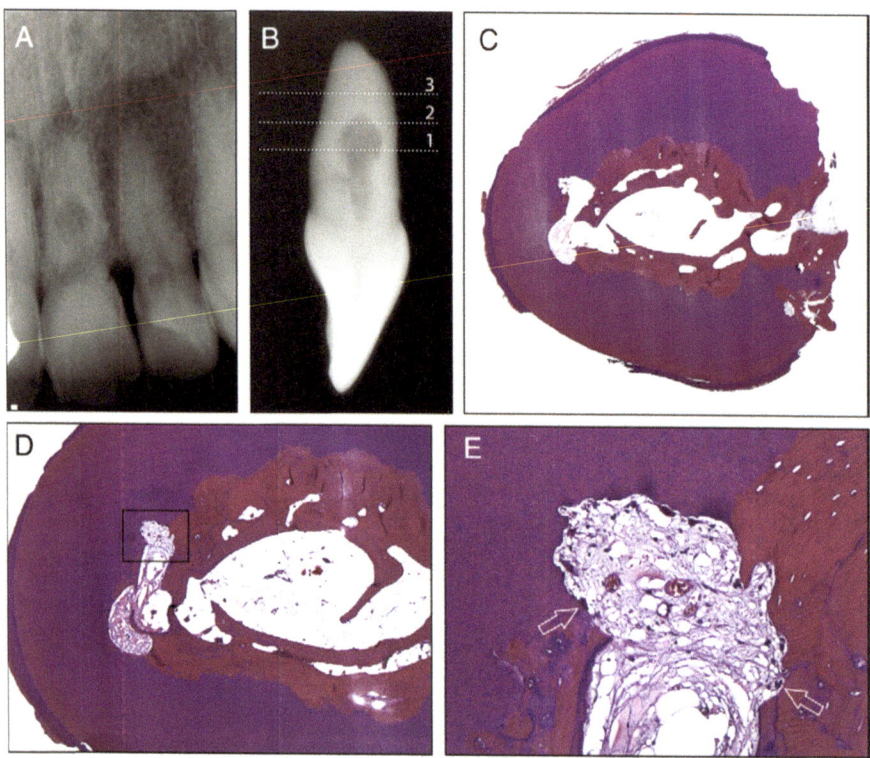

(a) Radiograph of a maxillary central incisor with a radiolucent lesion in the mid-third of the root canal suggestive of internal root resorption with metaplasia (b) Radiograph of the tooth after extraction showing the continuity of the resorptive lesion with the canal space (c) Cross section shows that the dentin around the root canal had been replaced by an ingrowth of bone tissue, and the root appears to have been perforated on the distopalatal aspect (d) Higher magnification of (c). (e) High magnification of the area demarcated by the rectangle in (d). The intraradicular dentin has been resorbed. (courtesy *Internal Root Resorption: A Review by* Dr.Shanon Patel)

Histologically, resorption of the intraradicular dentin is accompanied by subsequent deposition of a metaplastic hard tissue that resembles bone or cementum instead of dentin. Metaplasia refers to a reversible change in which one adult cell type (epithelial or mesenchymal) is replaced by another cell type. In the present context, the metaplastic tissue appears lamella-like, with entrapped osteocyte-like cells that resemble osteons of compact bone. A variant of internal root canal replacement resorption has previously been reported as "internal tunnelling resorption".

This entity is usually found in the coronal portion of root fractures but might also be seen after luxation injuries. The resorption process tunnels into the dentin adjacent to the root canal, with concomitant deposition of bonelike tissues in some regions. These bone-like tissues have the appearance of cancellous bone instead of compact bone. The process might subsequently arrest and might be followed by complete obliteration of the canal space by cancellous bone.[35]

HYPOTHESES REGARDING ORIGIN OF METAPLASTIC HARD TISSUES

The first hypothesis suggests that the metaplastic tissues are produced by postnatal dental pulp stem cells present in the apical, vital part of the root canal as a reparative response to the resorptive insult.[38] This is analogous to the formation of tertiary reparative dentin by odontoblast-like cells after the death of the primary odontoblasts. Unlike reactionary dentinogenesis, dentin repair studies have shown that the matrix deposited during reparative dentinogenesis demonstrates a high degree of heterogeneity. Following the depletion of epithelial-mesenchymal interactions that occur in primary dentinogenesis, the matrix deposited in reparative dentinogenesis often resembles osteoid instead of tubular dentin. Odontoblasts are postmitotic cells that are incapable of cell division following their terminal differentiation. In the absence of highly specific epigenetically derived signals required for lineage diversification and differentiation of "true" odontoblasts in an adult tooth, multipotent stem cells engaged in the process of reparative dentin formation retain the osteoblastic phenotype and secrete a matrix that more resembles bone than dentin.[39]

These histologic observations appear to be supported by the results of a recent article that involved the use of gene therapy to introduce a growth factor into dental pulp stem cells. In that study, the newly formed hard tissue resembled bone rather than dentin, with concentric lamellae of mineralized matrix entrapping osteocyte-like cells. In addition, a bone marrow–like hematopoietic tissue could be identified within the newly formed hard tissues. Thus, it is possible that a similar phenomenon occurs during the formation of metaplastic tissues in root canal replacement resorption.[40]

The second hypothesis proposes that both the granulation tissues and metaplastic hard tissues are of nonpulpal origin. Those tissues might be derived from cells that transmigrated from the vascular compartments or originated from the periodontium. This hypothesis suggests that in internal resorption, the pulpal tissues are replaced by periodontiumlike connective tissues.

Such a scenario is analogous to what occurs during ingrowth of connective tissues into the pulp space when a blood clot became available or, more recently, after pulpal revascularization procedures. Indeed, the histologic features of heavy inflammatory infiltrates and bone/cementum-like metaplastic tissues formation in root canal replacement resorption are highly reminiscent of similar unresolved lymphocyte infiltration and intracanal cementum-like hard tissue deposition in experimental revascularization procedures conducted in immature dog teeth with apical periodontitis.[41]

CLINICAL FEATURES OF INTERNAL RESORPTION

The clinical characteristics of internal root resorption are dependent on the development and location of the resorption. Most teeth with internal root resorption are symptom-free. However, when the resorption is actively progressing, the tooth is at least partially vital and may present symptoms typical of pulpitis. If the resorption occurs in or near the crown, it may in advanced cases show as a pinkish or reddish color through the crown if only a thin layer of enamel is left to cover the resorption.[42]

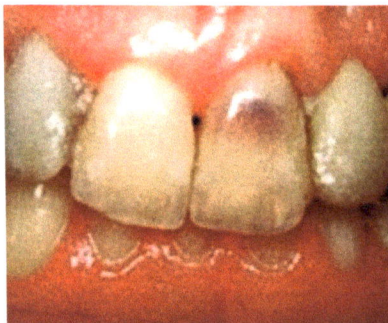
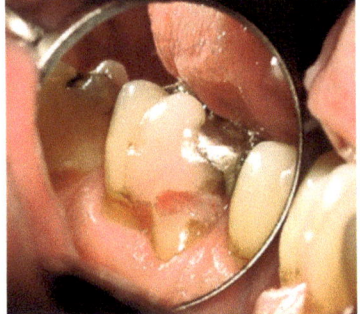

(courtesy Dr. M Hapaasalo)

The red color is caused by the highly vascularized connective tissue adjacent to the resorbing cells. Traditionally, the pink spot of Mummery has been thought to be pathognomonic of internal root resorption. However, these pink spots are also associated with external cervical resorptions. In internal resorption, the color is typically located centrally, whereas in cervical resorption the color ('pink spot') may also be mesially or distally located. Thus, differential diagnosis of internal root resorption cannot be based solely on the observation of pink spots. Teeth with untreated internal resorptions in the coronal area often turn gray/dark gray if the pulp becomes necrotic.[12]

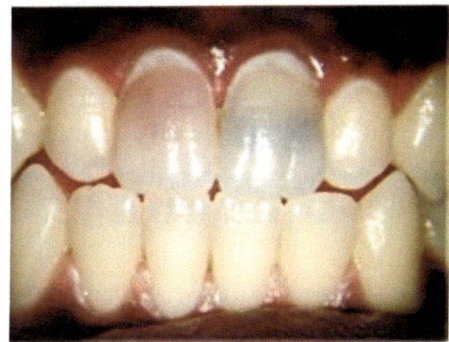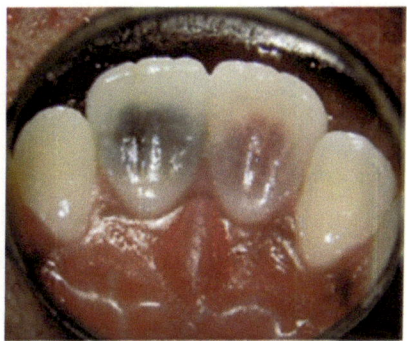

(Courtesy Dr. M. Ree)

Internal root resorptions continue to expand and eventually perforate the root until either endodontic treatment is started or the pulp becomes necrotic. Perforation of the root is usually followed by the development of a sinus tract, which confirms the presence of an infection in the root canal. After the perforation, the continuation of the resorption may no longer be dependent on the presence of vital pulp tissue because the resorbing cells may now obtain nutrients from tissues surrounding the tooth. After perforation, the control of infection is more difficult than in an unperforated root canal. The tooth structure is also weaker in teeth with perforation as a result of loss of hard tissue. In addition to the sinus tract, swelling may be present, while most patients complain of only mild or no pain.[43]

With advancing infection, the entire pulp becomes necrotic and internal root resorption ceases because the resorbing cells are cut off from the circulation and nutrients, unless root perforation has occurred before the development of total necrosis. Pulpal necrosis can therefore be regarded as an effective protection against spreading of the resorption. The consequence of pulp necrosis is, as usual, apical periodontitis.

RADIOGRAPHIC FEATURES OF INTERNAL RESORPTION

Internal root resorption is relatively easy to identify radiographically and is seen as a radiolucent, round and symmetrical widening of the root canal space. At the area of the resorption, the original canal shape can no longer be observed. However, not all internal root resorptions show similar progression, and oval as well as asymmetrically shaped internal root resorptions can be found. In the coronal pulp/ crown area, internal resorption can be symmetrical in teeth with one root canal and a narrow pulp chamber where pulp horns are situated close to each other. However, in molar teeth with several roots and a wide pulp chamber, internal resorption may begin at one part of the chamber and spread locally into the surrounding dentin. In such cases, it may be difficult to make the diagnosis between internal and external cervical resorption until the resorptive area is accessed directly, cleaned and carefully studied under a surgical microscope during endodontic treatment.However, cervical resorptions in the crown area often have a more irregular outline and contain randomly shaped thin opaque lines which are not seen in lesions of internal resorption.[44]

The problem in diagnosis occurs when the external cervical resorption lesion is not accessible by probing and is projected radiologically over the root canal. Both lesions might have a similar radiographic appearance. Gartner et al described guidelines that enable clinicians to differentiate the two processes radiographically. The authors reported internal root resorption lesions to be smooth and generally symmetrically distributed over the root. They described the radiolucency of the internal root resorption as having a uniform density. The pulp chamber or root canal outline could not be followed through the lesion, because the canal walls essentially balloon out.[45] Internal root resorption lesions might also be oval, circumscribed radiolucencies in continuity with the canal walls. Lesions caused by external cervical lesion, by contrast, have borders that are ill-defined and asymmetrical, with radiodensity variations in the body of the lesion.[46]

The canal wall should be traceable through the external cervical resorption lesion because the latter is superimposed over the root canal. The use of parallax radiographic techniques is advocated for differentiating internal from external resorption defects. A second radiograph taken at a different angle often confirms the nature of the resorptive lesion. ECR lesions will move in the same direction as the x-ray tube shift if they are lingually/palatally positioned. They will move in the opposite direction to the tube shift if they are buccally positioned. Conversely, internal root resorption lesions should remain in the same position relative to the canal in both radiographs.[47] Radiologically, internal replacement resorption presents as a cloudy, mottled, radiopaque lesion with irregular margins as a result of the presence of metaplastic hard tissue deposits within the canal space. Differentiating internal replacement resorption from external cervical resorption might be clinically challenging,especially if the metaplasia has occupied the entire resorptive cavity.[48]

The advent of cone beam computed tomography (CBCT) has enhanced radiographic diagnosis. The use of CBCT provides greater 3-dimensional geometric accuracy when compared with conventional radiography.[32] The use of CBCT can be invaluable in the decision-making process. The scanned data provide the clinician with a 3-dimensional appreciation of the tooth, the resorption lesion, and the adjacent anatomy. The true nature of the lesion might be assessed, including root perforations and whether the lesion is amendable to treatment.[49]

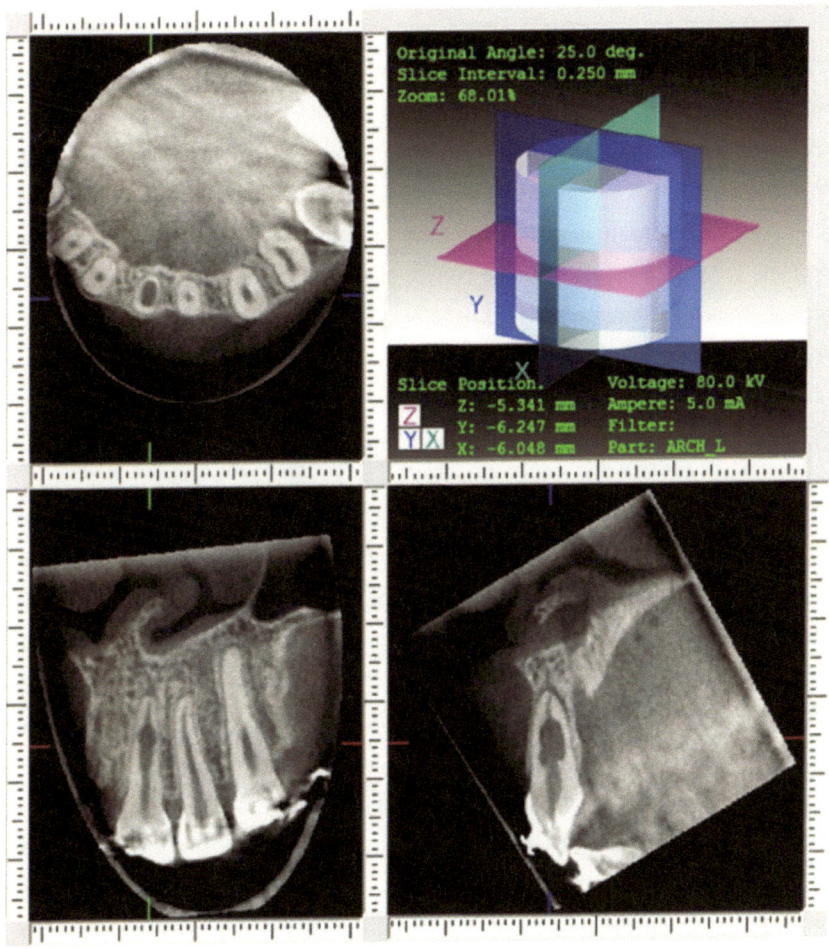

(Courtesy of Drs. T. Cotton, T. Geisler, D. Holden, S. Schwartz, and W. Schindler)

TREATMENT PERSPECTIVES

Once internal root resorption has been diagnosed, the clinician must make a decision on the prognosis of the tooth. If the tooth is deemed restorable and has a reasonable prognosis, root canal treatment is the treatment of choice. The aim of root canal treatment is to remove any remaining vital, apical tissue and the necrotic coronal portion of the pulp that might be sustaining and stimulating the resorbing cells via their blood supply, and to disinfect and obturate the root canal system. Internal root resorption lesions present the endodontist with unique difficulties in the preparation and obturation of the affected tooth.[50] Access cavity preparation should be conservative, preserving as much tooth structure as possible, and should avoid further weakening of the already compromised tooth. In teeth with actively resorbing lesions, bleeding from the inflamed pulpal and granulation tissues might be profuse and might impair visibility during the initial stages of chemomechanical debridement. The shape of the resorption defect usually renders it inaccessible to direct mechanical instrumentation.[52]

INSTRUMENTATION OF TEETH WITH INTERNAL RESORPTION

Instrumentation and cleaning of the root canal space of teeth with internal esorption faces a few challenges different from those of normal endodontic treatment. In cases where the resorption is active, there is typically brisk bleeding from the pulp tissue, which may make it difficult to locate the root canal openings. However, as soon as the apical pulp tissue has been cut off and removed using large enough instruments in the apical canal, the bleeding stops or is greatly reduced, allowing better visibility into the work area.[11] Irrigation by concentrated sodium hypochlorite will in most cases help to reduce the bleeding. Sometimes it is preferable to pack calcium hydroxide into the pulp chamber and the canal and seal the tooth with a temporary filling. A few days later, bleeding of the soft tissue is no longer a problem because calcium hydroxide effectively necrotizes the granulation tissue. For teeth where the resorption has perforated the root, placement of calcium hydroxide is recommended to necrotize the resorptive tissue and to stop the bleeding.[53]

Although the majority of the literature on internal root resorption is case reports, there is no generally accepted protocol for the chemomechanical instrumentation of the root canal system in these cases. However, it is obvious that a great emphasis must be placed on the chemical dissolution of the vital and necrotic pulp tissue. Therefore, irrigation with sodium hypochlorite is an important part of the treatment of teeth with internal resorption. Small perforations do not seem to require abandonment of the use of hypochlorite; on the contrary, hypochlorite will help to control bleeding from the perforation and disinfect the area as experienced with accidental perforation complications. However, with large perforations, low-concentration hypochlorite solutions should be used and other irrigants such as chlorhexidine should be considered.[54] The shape of a resorbed root canal prevents instrument access to all areas of the canal. Creating a straight line access to the resorption cannot be done in many cases because it would weaken the tooth structure too much. This is one reason why the use of ultrasound has been advocated for the treatment of internal resorptions. Ultrasound can facilitate the penetration of an irrigant to all areas of the root canal system and break loose necrotic tissue in the canal. In order to better reach the most distant areas of the resorption, hand instruments are often bent at 1–4mm from the tip to help to gain contact with the walls of the resorption cavity and help to remove all soft tissue. Although use of hypochlorite and ultrasound are mainly responsible for cleaning of the most challenging areas, the importance of careful mechanical cleaning should not be underestimated.[55]

INTRACANAL MEDICAMENTS FOR INTERNAL RESORPTION

Intracanal interappointment medicaments are used in endodontic treatments mainly to maximize the effect of disinfection procedures. In the treatment of internal resorption, the use of calcium hydroxide also has two other important goals: to control bleeding, and to necrotize residual pulp tissue and to make the necrotic tissue more soluble to sodium hypochlorite. Because of the limited access by instruments to all areas of the resorption cavity, chemical means are needed to completely clean the canal. Studies Morgan et al. on the effectiveness of sodium hypochlorite and calcium hydroxide to remove the resorptive and other tissues from the root canal indicate that they have an additive or even synergistic effect. In cases where the resorption has not perforated, it is usually enough to use calcium hydroxide paste in the canal once from 1 to 2 weeks. This allows removal of the residual tissue at the next appointment by irrigation and instrumentation.[44]

Ultrasound is recommended both to facilitate tissue removal and for cleaning the canal from all calcium hydroxide before permanent root filling. In perforated internal resorptions, calcium hydroxide treatment has been carried out for extended time periods for up to 1 year to secure complete healing of the site of perforation. There are no comparative studies on the long-term prognosis of perforated internal resorptions treated with either short-term or long-term calcium hydroxide treatment. However, it is possible that the new material, mineral trioxide aggregate (MTA), could change the recommended treatment protocol for internal resorption.

A number of recent studies, including two meta-analyses by Peng et al and Aeinehchi et al, have shown that MTA is superior to formocresol in pulpotomies of primary molars. A notable difference between the two materials was the absence of resorption complications following treatment in the MTA groups.[28] Recently, filling of the internal resorption cavity with MTA in a primary molar was reported by Sonmenz et al. Although not supported yet by long-term results from clinical studies, it is possible that the treatment of perforated internal resorptions in the future will consist of a thorough chemomechanical cleaning and disinfection of the root canal and resorption area including the perforation site, followed by a short-term calcium hydroxide treatment. At the second appointment, in the absence of any clinical symptoms, the resorption cavity will be filled with MTA.[45]

PERMANENT FILLING OF ROOT CANAL AND INTERNAL RESORPTION

There is no generally accepted consensus on the materials and techniques that should be given priority when teeth with internal resorptions are permanently filled. However, case reports and clinical experience indicate that root filling methods using warm gutta-percha are generally preferred over other techniques. However, in cases where the resorption has perforated, MTA should be considered instead of gutta-percha because of its antimicrobial properties and better seal. MTA is also very well tolerated by the tissues. MTA carriers, ultrasound, inverted paper points used as pluggers, and radiographic control of the MTA filling at the early phase of condensation are all crucial factors for success and to ensure a high quality filling. In teeth with a large resorption cavity in the coronal third of the root canal, use of composite materials should be considered in order to strengthen the tooth and to make it more resistant to fracture.[46]

TREATMENT

Initial phase (Preventive phase):

1. Prevention of the initial injury

Usage of mouth-guards, face shields and other protective devices

2. Minimizing Additional Damage after the Injury

- In case of luxations, gentle repositioning of the tooth in its original position can be done.
- In case of splinting, functional splint for 7-10 days and splint should be constructed to allow adequate cleaning.

3. Pharmacological manipulation of initial inflammatory response

- The drugs that affects osteoclasts present at the site of resorption are: Tetracyclines
- The drugs that affect the recruitment of osteoclasts to the injury site are:

    -Glucocorticoids eg. Topical dexamethasone

    -Bisphoshonates eg. Alendronate

Secondary phase:

1. Prevention of pulp space infection

Maintain the vitality of the pulp

Aims at promoting revascularization of the pulp space in severe injuries where vitality is lost.

Indicated in teeth with incompletely formed apices, where > 1.1 mm wide radiographically.

However, the disadvantages of revascularization are:

-Even under the best conditions revascularization will occur only in less than 50% of the cases.

-Risk of inflammatory resorption and rapid loss of tooth structure due to large dentinal tubules and thin dentinal walls of immature teeth.(Bakland 1992)

2. Elimination of pulp space infection

Indicated when root canal treatment initiated later than 10 days after the accident and there is presence of active external inflammatory resorption.

Application of intracanal medications

Calcium hydroxide: Increases the pH of dentin by inhibiting the activity of osteoclastic acid hydrolases in the periodontal tissues and activates alkaline phosphatases. It has a lasting antibacterial activity with low solubility and inactivation of endotoxin (Leonardo et al 2004)

Disadvantages includes unsatisfactory permeability of hydroxyl ions through dentinal tubules, low solubility and long term use could reduce the fracture resistance of tooth.

Iodine potassium iodine (IKI) + Calcium hydroxide: have improved penetration and are more soluble. Disadvantages are allergic reaction to iodine and short duration of antimicrobial action.

Electrophoretically activated copper+ Calcium hydroxide: Improved penetration but disadvantages are tooth discoloration from the copper and periapical toxicity.(Fuss et al 2002)

Electrophoretically activated calcium hydroxide: Properties are strong antibacterial effect in dentinal tubules, better penetration, eliminates viable bacteria in shorter time.(Tsesis et al 2005)

Activ Point (Activ point, Roeko, Langenau, Germany): Contains 5% chlorhexidine diacetate and has shown significantly stronger antibacterial effect in dentinal tubules to a depth of 500μm compared to calcium hydroxide or irrigation with chlorhexidine alone.

3. Manipulation of the inflammatory response

-Ledermix

•Drug combining tetracycline (demethylchlortetracycline) and corticosteroid (triamcinolone acetonide) and has a synergistic effect on the inhibition of root resorption.

•It eliminates pulp space infection as well as suppresses inflammation.

-Calcitonin

- It is a polypeptide hormone.
- Resorbing cells are the only cells that have receptors for calcitonin.
- Use has been proposed in an attempt to control the resorption process

-Bisphoshonateseg. Alendronate

-Amino acids eg. Taurine

CHAPTER 5: EXTERNAL ROOT RESORPTION

External root resorption is a much more difficult condition to diagnose and manage. It has been described by a variety of names, which may describe the location, etiology, or pathogenesis of the lesion. External resorption may be caused by physical damage to the external protective layer of precementum; by trauma, infection, or both. In certain cases, the etiology is of unknown origin. External root resorption can be further classified into surface resorption, external inflammatory resorption, external replacement resorption, external cervical resorption and transient apical breakdown.[47]

DIFFERENCE BETWEEN INTERNAL AND EXTERNAL ROOT RESORPTION

INTERNAL ROOT RESORPTION	*EXTERNAL ROOT RESORPTION*
The margins are smooth and clearly defined	The borders may be ill defined
Their distribution over the root is symmetrical but may be eccentric	Their distribution is not symmetrical and may occur on any root surface
The radiolucency is of uniform density	There may be variations in radiodensity in the body of the lesion
The pulp chamber or canal cannot be followed through the lesion	If the lesion is superimposed on the root canal system, it should be possible to follow the canal walls unaltered through the area of the defect
The walls of the root canal system may appear to balloon out	There is no alteration in the root canal system

EXTERNAL SURFACE RESORPTION

It is small, superficial resorption cavities in the cementum and the outermost layers of the dentin, without an inflammatory reaction in the periodontal ligament[16] Andreason & Hansen (1966)

Etiology:

☐ Indirect physical injury to periodontal ligament or cementum

☐ Certain cases of trauma which results in direct mechanical contact of root surface and alveolar bone proper

Clinical Features:

It is a normal physiologic response according to Ne et al. It is commonly associated with normal turnover of cementum and is considered a transient and self limiting phenomenon as there is spontaneous destruction and repair which occurs within 2-3 weeks. It is considered the least destructive form of external resorption. Usually there is no significant signs of external surface resorption detectable on the supragingival portion of the tooth.[7]

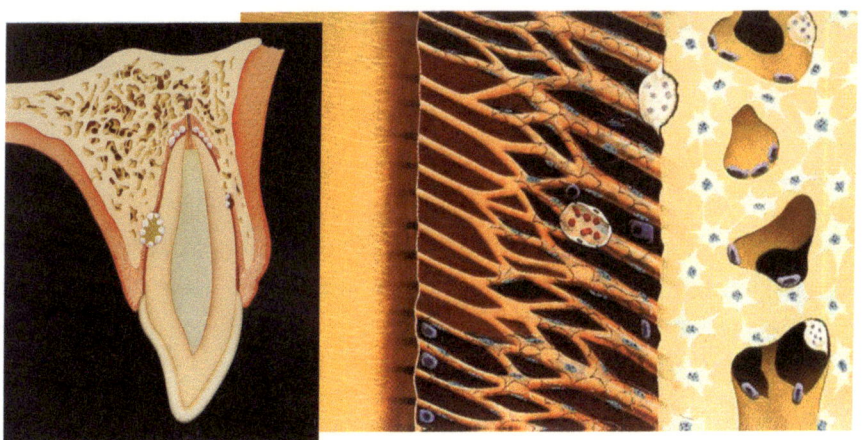

(Courtesy Dr.Zvi Fuss)

Radiographic evaluation:

External surface resorption is usually not visible on radiographs. Rarely seen as small excavations on root surface with normal lamina dura and periodontal space.

Histologic evaluation:

☐ Small, superficial lacunae in the cementum and the outermost layer of dentin

☐ Repair with cementum like tissue

☐ Generally no significant inflammatory reaction in the adjacent periodontal ligament

Treatment:

Usually the condition is asymptomatic and no treatment is indicated as it is a self limiting condition.

EXTERNAL CERVICAL RESORPTION

External cervical resorption is the loss of dental hard tissue as a result of odontoclastic action; it usually begins on the cervical region of the root surface of the teeth. ECR usually occurs immediately below the epithelial attachment of the tooth at the cervical region. ECR defects can be difficult to diagnose and manage.

Synonyms for external cervical resorption are: *Invasive cervical resorption, odontoclastoma, peripheral cervical resorption, extracanal invasive resorption, supraosseous extracanal invasive resorption, peripheral inflammatory root resorption and subepithelial external root resorption.*[48]

Etiology:

The exact cause of ECR is poorly understood. Several predisposing factors have been suggested that might damage the cervical region of the root surface and therefore initiate ECR. These include the following:

- ❖ Dental trauma
- ❖ Orthodontic treatment
- ❖ Intracoronal bleaching
- ❖ Periodontal therapy
- ❖ Idiopathic

Trauma: ECR is a recognized complication of luxation and avulsion injuries. Heithersay confirmed that dental trauma was a major potential predisposing factor for ECR. Dental trauma can also cause ECR indirectly. Intruded primary incisors might cause developmental defects in the cervical region on the unerupted permanent successor teeth as a result of direct trauma of the root apices on the unerupted successor. The use of splints (especially interdental wiring) might also potentially damage the cementoenamel junction and therefore predispose to ECR.

Orthodontic Treatment: Excessive orthodontic forces at the cervical region of the tooth might result in tissue necrosis adjacent to exposed root dentin. This might result in mononuclear precursor cells being stimulated to differentiate into odontoclasts, which are attracted to and resorb the exposed root dentin. Heithersay found that the most commonly affected teeth were maxillary canines, maxillary incisors, and mandibular molars.

Intracoronal Bleaching: Heithersay reported intracoronal bleaching as a sole and associated predisposing factor for ECR in 3.9% and 13.6% of cases, respectively. Several suggestions have been put forward for the actual mechanism by which intracoronal bleaching might result in ECR. Rotstein et al. demonstrated that the presence of cemental defects at the cementoenamel junction could result in hydrogen peroxide from the pulp chamber of root-filled teeth escaping to the external tooth surface via dentinal tubules during intracoronal bleaching with 30% hydrogen peroxide. It has been suggested that hydrogen peroxide might denature dentin and provoke an immunologic response. In addition, the pH at the root surface of teeth is reduced to about 6.5 by intracoronal placement of a "walking bleach" paste. This slightly acidic environment is known to enhance osteoclastic activity, which might result in ECR.[49]

Periodontal Therapy: Unexpectedly, periodontal debridement that might inadvertently result in damage/removal of the cementum was not identified in the study by Heithersay as a major predisposing factor. Periodontal therapy was recorded as the sole predisposing factor in only 1.6% of patients. The incidence appeared to be consistently low, even when combined with other factors. ECR might be prevented after periodontal debridement of the root surface by rapid epithelial down growth preventing contact of connective tissue cells with that surface, thus hindering the inflammatory process. Ben-Yehouda described a case of ECR that had previously been treated with tetracycline root-conditioning.

Other Factors: Other factors that have been suggested as potential predisposing factors to ECR include bruxism and intracoronal restorations. Developmental defects such as hypoplasia or hypomineralization of cementum have also been suggested as predisposing factors.

Diagnosis:

ECR is usually found at the cervical region of the tooth. A pink spot in the cervical region of the tooth is usually the clinical sign noticed by the patient and/or dentist that brings the problem to light. This discoloration is a result of the highly vascular granulation (resorptive) tissue within the tooth becoming visible through the thinned out (resorbed) dentin and translucent overlying enamel.

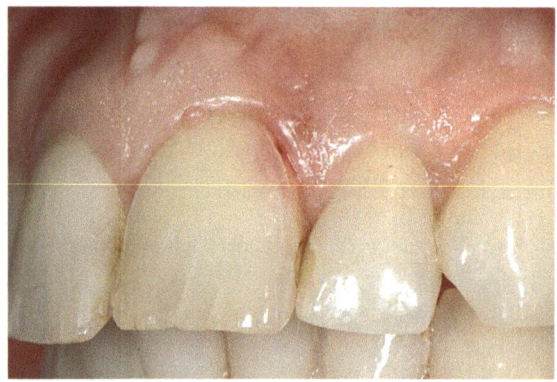

Pink spot and a probable defect on the distal aspect in the cervical region of the maxillary left central incisor, indicating ECR.(courtesy Dr.Shanon Patel)

It is important to differentiate ECR from subgingival caries, which will feel sticky on probing and does not present with the pink spot. The base of an ECR defect will feel hard and also result in a scraping sound when probed. Probing the ECR defect and/or the associated periodontal pocket will cause profuse bleeding of the underlying highly vascular resorptive tissue. Once the granulation tissue has been removed from an ECR lesion, the cavity walls will feel hard and mineralized on probing. The edges of the cavity usually appear sharp and narrow. Teeth with ECR will respond positively to sensitivity testing because the pulp only becomes involved in very advanced cases of ECR.[45]

Early ECR defects are commonly detected as chance findings on radiographs. The severity of ECR determines its radiographic appearance. The lesion classically presents as an asymmetrical radiolucency with ragged or irregular margins in the cervical region of the tooth.

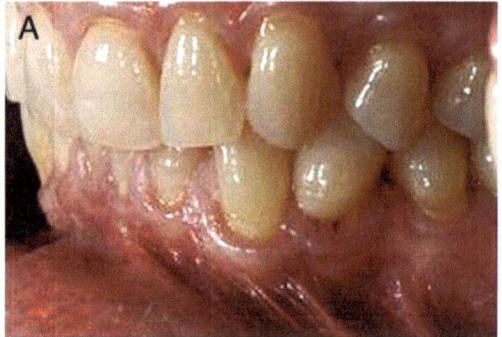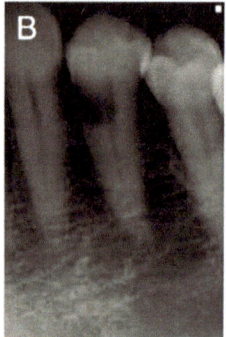

(A) Probable defect is detected on the buccal cervical aspect of the mandibular left first premolar. (B) Radiograph reveals a radiolucent lesion with poorly defined borders, indicating the lesion is ECR.(courtesy Dr.Shanon Patel)

Early lesions might be radiolucent; however, more advanced lesions might have a mottled appearance caused by the osseous nature of the advanced lesion. The outline of the root canal should be visible and intact, indicating that the lesion lies on the outer surface of the root. With more advanced lesions, the lesion tends to balloon out within the root in all directions; this will also be reflected in the size and position of the radiolucency detected on the radiograph. The lesion might involve the adjacent alveolus, resulting in a radiographic appearance of an intrabony defect.[27] The parallax technique is useful to follow the continuity of the pulp canal and to distinguish between internal and external resorption. With internal resorption, the defect remains centered on the root canal system regardless of the angle of the radiograph exposure, whereas with ECR the defect will either move in the same (lingual/palatal) or in the opposite (labial) direction of the x-ray tube. The radiologic appearance of ECR does not always follow this classic appearance. It might vary from a round, uniformly radiolucent lesion with well-defined smooth symmetrical borders to a multiloculated lesion with a mottled appearance.[60]

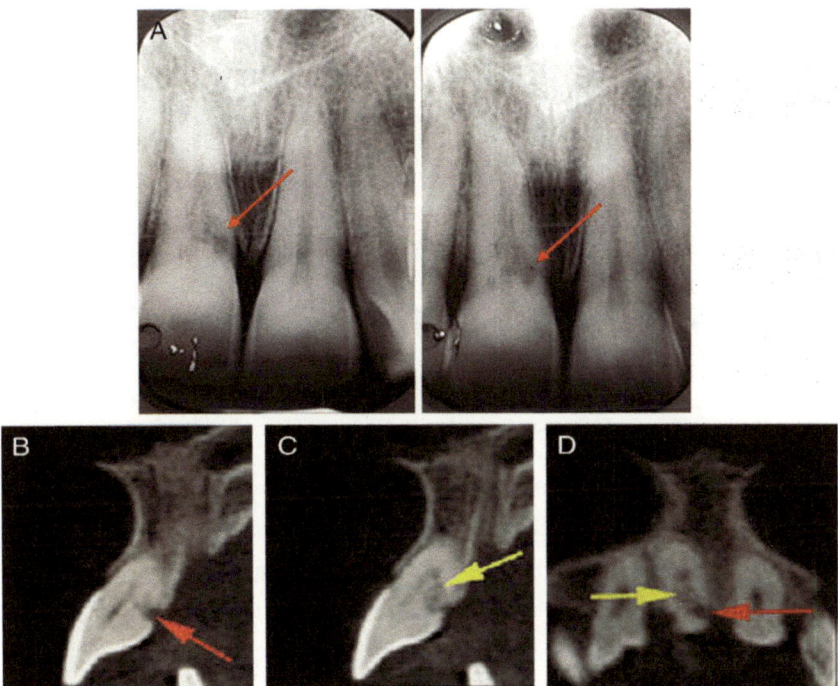

(A) Two periapical radiographs made at different horizontal angles confirm the resorptive lesion is palatally positioned by using the parallax principle. The lesion appears to extend mesially, although this is difficult to confirm. (B, C) A series of CBCT sagittal slices and (D) an axial view clearly show 2 distinct areas within the resorptive lesion: outer inflammatory (red arrow) and an inner fibro-osseous (yellow arrow) resorption. Int Endod J 2007; 40:818–830.

A distinction must also be made between early ECR and cervical "burnout," which might appear as a radiolucent band across the entire neck of the tooth. It has been shown that conventional radiographic techniques reveal limited information on the true extent and nature of the resorptive lesion. Recently, cone beam computed tomography (CBCT), which is an extraoral 3-dimensional imaging technique, has been used to assess ECR lesions. The position, depth in relation to the root canal, and ultimately the restorability of the tooth can be assessed objectively before any treatment is carried out.[44]

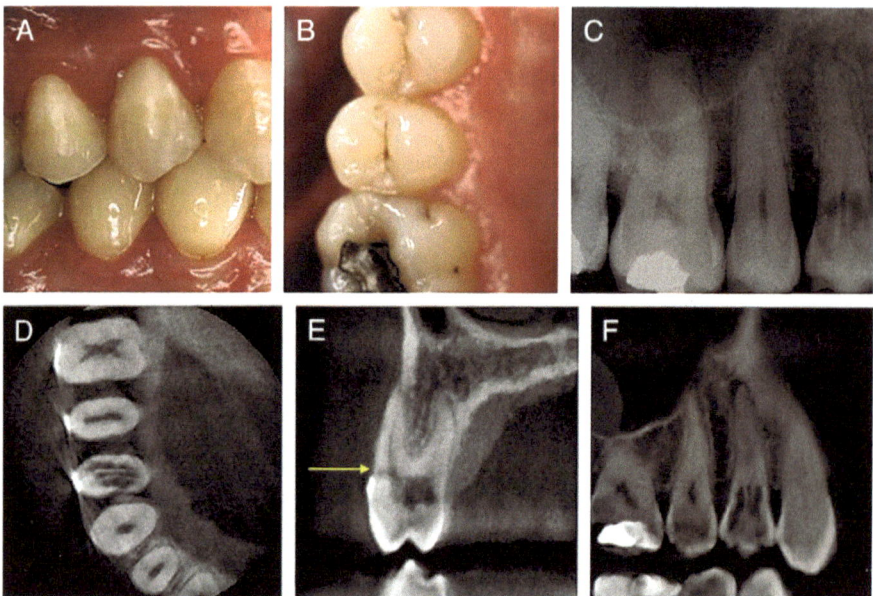

(A, B) Clinical views of the maxillary right quadrant. Note there are no clinical signs of ECR. (C) A periapical radiograph reveals extensive ECR. (D–F) With CBCT the true nature of the lesion can be established, including the portal of entry (yellow arrow).(courtesy Dr.Shanon Patel)

Atypical internal resorption lesions located on the outer aspects of the root canal might also be confused with ECR. As a result of the internal resorption lesion not being located centrally, the root canal might still be visible on a conventional radiograph, and the parallax principle might confuse matters more because the lesion will move with the changing position of the tube head.[12]

HISTOLOGIC FEATURES

The resorptive cavity in ECR lesions consists of granulomatous tissue. Osteoclasts might be observed on the resorbing front within the lacunae. The predentin and innermost layer of dentin prevent the ECR lesion from involving the pulp, which remains healthy (uninflamed) until the ECR has become very advanced. Resorption channels extend into the dentin and interconnect within the periodontal ligament. As the lesion advances, bone-like material might also become deposited within the lesion and also in direct contact with the adjacent dentin.[51]

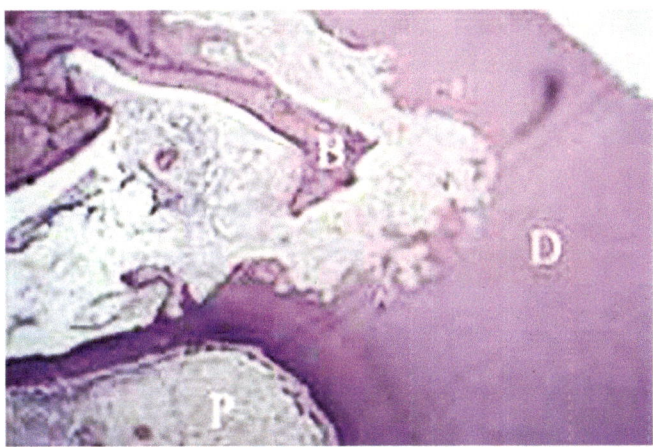

Figure 8. Horizontal histologic section of ECR shows bone (B) forming within the dentin (D). The resorptive process avoids the dentin that surrounds the pulp. (courtesy Dr.Pitt Ford T)

The advancing ECR lesions characteristically stop short of the root canal and underlying pulp; instead, the resorptive process usually expands in a circumferential and apico-coronal direction around the root canal. Perforation of the root canal is prevented by a thin protective layer of inner dentin and predentin. The predentin has been shown to contain an anti-invasion factor and resorption inhibitor that prevent ECR from advancing into the root canal until the ECR is very advanced. It has also been suggested that the outer surface of enamel might also be resistant to resorption as a result of preferential odontoclastic dissolution of interprismatic enamel.Early ECR defects do not usually contain acute inflammatory cells, implying a nonbacterial etiology. However, at a later stage, a secondary bacterial colonization of dentinal tubules might induce an inflammatory response in the associated periodontal or pulpal tissue. In long-standing lesions, the root canal might be perforated by the advancing resorptive lesion. If pulpal involvement occurs, the fibroosseous tissue can be found deposited within the root canal system.[52]

Treatment:

Treatment depends on the severity, location, whether the defect has perforated the root canal system, and the restorability of the tooth. Several treatment regimes have been suggested depending on the nature of the ECR lesion which includes:

- ❖ Intentional replantation
- ❖ Guided tissue regeneration
- ❖ Treating the ECR lesion by an internal approach
- ❖ Treating the ECR lesion by an external approach
- ❖ Forced orthodontic eruption

The aim of treatment should be to:

▶ Stop continuation of resorption by removing all the granulomatous tissue from the root. In cases where removal of granulomatous tissue would cause unacceptable damage to supporting structures, an attempt is made to sever the blood supply to the granulomatous tissue, thus killing the resorptive cells and inhibiting progression of the resorptive process

▶ Replace the unprotected root surface with a foreign material that clastic cells cannot be attached to or penetrate, such as any well-sealing dental restorative material.

Essentially, treatment involves complete removal of the resorptive tissue and restoring the resulting defect with a plastic tooth-colored restoration. Endodontic treatment might also be required in cases in which the ECR lesion has perforated the root canal.

External Approach

Determine the exact location of the defect (buccal or lingual-palatal) using angled radiographs .A full thickness flap is raised and granulomatous tissue is removed from the root and the bone defect with a curette or bur. Also remove granulomatous tissue from sound, healthy bone so that revascularization of the resorbing tissues will not occur. The opening into the root should be as conservative as possible. The root defect is filled with a restorative material and the flap is replaced in a way as to minimize the periodontal defect after healing. It is mostly indicated for the small coronal defect.[45]

Internal Approach

▶ trichloracetic acid: the acid will chemically burn the granulomatous tissue, thus necrosing it and providing space for the filling material internally

▶ calcium hydroxide: it may take multiple applications to achieve the same results

Theoretically, a bur could be used but the chances of pulp exposure and/or extensive attachment damage are very high with this approach

Combined approach

Elective endodontic therapy is often the best choice in extensive lesions. A flap is raised and the granulomatous tissue is aggressively removed from the bony defect. A barrier membrane is used to stop new tissue from growing into the root and to stop revascularization of the necrotic tissue left inside the root. After approximately one month, an opening is made externally above the attachment and the necrotic granulomatous tissue is removed and replaced with a filling material such as mineral trioxide aggregate.

Forced eruption: This is advocated if the remaining root apical to the resorption defect is long enough to maintain the tooth. The resorption defect is moved to a position coronal to the adjacent attachment. Later the defect is cleaned and restored.

Intentional replantation: This is executed if the practitioner is confident that the resorbed root will not fracture on extraction.

EXTERNAL INFLAMMATORY RESORPTION

This type of resorption was described in a clinical and histologic study of avulsed and replanted teeth by Andreasen et al. in 1965. It is an infection related resorption which represents a combined injury to the pulp and periodontal ligament and where bacteria, primarily located in the pulp space and in the dentinal tubules, triggers osteoclastic activity on the root surface. This type of resorption can affect all parts of root.[26] It is exclusively related to acute trauma and is especially common after intrusion and replantation of avulsed teeth.

Clinical Findings:

The tooth undergoing infection-related root resorption will have increased mobility and have a dull percussion tone. Sometimes the tooth may be extruded. Sensitivity tests gives no response, and sometimes a sinus tract develops.

Radiographic Findings:

Infection-related resorption is typically diagnosed 2-4 weeks after injury and appears as progressive cavitations involving the root and adjacent alveolar bone. The resorption is rapidly progressing event that may result in total loss of root structure after only a few months, particularly in young children.

Treatment:

The treatment goal is to remove or destroy bacteria in the root canal and dentinal tubules to allow healing to take place in the entire periradicular space. The bacteria are best destroyed by using calcium hydroxide as an intracanal medicament. However, a side effect of using calcium hydroxide for a long term i.e more than 30 days is weakening of the root structure in immature teeth;this may lead to cervical root fractures. This is a risk that has been found to be as high as 66-72%. In mature teeth, the problem apparently does not exist. The endodontic technique therefore varies according to the maturity of the tooth.

In fully developed teeth with inflammatory resorption, endodontic treatment should include prophylactic extirpation of the pulp space in replanted avulsed teeth. Biomechanical canal preparation should include the use of sodium hypochlorite and calcium hydroxide. The latter can be expected to have accomplished its task of disinfection so that the canal can be filled 2-3 weeks after treatment[4]

In situations in which the pulp becomes necrotic before the root is fully developed, the apical opening is often too large to create a resistance to retain the root canal filling. Apexification procedures using calcium hydroxide have been performed with good success. The disadvantage of using calcium hydroxide for apexification is that it takes many months to obtain enough barrier to allow placement of a root canal filling. Additionally, it appears that long term use of calcium hydroxide can weaken dentin, possibly by dissolving its organic component and thereby resulting in cervical root fracture on even slight impacts or normal use. By using MTA as a physical barrier apically, a root canal filling can be placed immediately without waiting for a biological response. Minimizing exposure of root dentin to calcium hydroxide results in less damage to the dentin.[16] It is to be understood that dentin lost through resorption cannot be replaced by new dentin. Healing occurs by arresting the resorption process and replacement with either a layer of new cementum or bone and establishment of new periodontal ligament.

INITIAL PHASE (PREVENTIVE PHASE)

1. Prevention of the initial injury

- ▶ usage of mouth-guards, face shields and other protective devices

2. Minimizing Additional Damage after the Injury

- ▶ Luxations
    - Gentle repositioning of the tooth in its original position
    - Splinting
        - ▶ functional splint for 7-10 days
        - ▶ splint should be constructed to allow adequate cleaning

3. Pharmacological manipulation of the initial inflammatory response

- ▶ Drugs that affects osteoclasts present at the site of resorption
    - Tetracyclines
        - ▶ Sustained antimicrobial effect
        - ▶ Anti-resorptive properties
            - direct inhibitory effect on osteoclasts and collagenase
        - ▶ Significantly more cemental healing
- ▶ Drugs that affect the recruitment of osteoclasts to the injury site
    - Glucocorticoids
        - ▶ Topical dexamethasone

- Bisphoshonates [20,21]
    - ▶ Alendronate
    - ▶ Can inhibit bone resorption in several ways:
        - inhibiting osteoblast-induced recruitment of osteoclasts to bone resorption sites
        - inhibiting osteoclast activity upon cell contact with bisphosphonates
        - premature apoptosis (or cell-destruction) of osteoclasts
- Amino acids [20]
    - ▶ Taurine
        - α amino acid
        - Inhibits PGE2 and IL-1 mediated osteoclast formation
- ▶ Combination of the two types of drugs
    - synergistic effect on the inhibition of root resorption
    - Ledermix [22, 23]
        - ▶ a drug combining tetracycline (demethylchlortetracycline) and corticosteroid (trimcinolone acetonide)
- ▶ ART (Antiresorptive Regenerative Therpay) [9] *by Pohl et al 2005*
    - Comprises a combination of different treatment strategies for a synergistic effect
        - ▶ Local application of a glucocorticoid
        - ▶ Systemic and local application of tetracyclines
        - ▶ Use of Enamel Matrix Derivative (EMD) e.g. Emdogain

4. Stimulate Cemental Healing

- ▶ 'Conditioned Medium'
    - supernatant of cultured gingival fibroblasts, that contain a number of biologically active factors
- ▶ ViaSpan

- ▶ Emdogain (Enamel Matrix Protein; Biora, Malmo, Sweden)
    - for teeth with extended extra oral dry times
    - makes the root more resistant to resorption
    - stimulates the formation of new periodontal ligament from the socket

5. Slow down 'inevitable' osseous replacement

- ▶ When the periodontal ligament on the root surface is definitely destroyed
    - intrusive injuries
    - avulsion injuries with extended extra-oral dry times
- ▶ Intrusive injuries
    - the tooth is repositioned
    - inevitable osseous replacement accepted
- ▶ Avulsion injuries with extended dry times [8]
    - All remaining periodontal ligament debris is removed from the root by thorough curettage
    - Fluoride
        - ▶ root is soaked in fluoride for 5 min before replantation
        - ▶ effectively slow down remodeling of the root to bone
    - Bisphosphonates
        - ▶ slows down the osseous replacement
        - ▶ More expensive than fluoride
    - Emdogain

SECONDARY PHASE (TREATMENT PHASE)

1. Prevention of pulp space infection [26, 27]

- A) Maintain the vitality of the pulp
    - Aims at promoting revascularization of the pulp space in severe injuries where vitality is lost

B) Prevent root canal infection by root canal treatment at 7-10 days

- Teeth with closed apices

    ▶ When trauma is severe

    ▶ Treat within 7-10 days of the injury before the ischemically necrosed pulp becomes infected

2. *Elimination of pulp space infection*

▶ **Indicated**

- When root canal treatment initiated later than 10 days after the accident
- Presence of active external inflammatory resorption

▶ **Use of intracanal medications**

- Calcium hydroxide
- Iodine potassium iodine (IKI)
- Electrophoretically activated copper
- Electrophoretically activated calcium hydroxide
- Activ Point (Activ point, Roeko, Langenau, Germany)

3. *Manipulation of the inflammatory response*

- *Ledermix:* A drug combining tetracycline (demethylchlortetracycline) and corticosteroid (trimcinolone acetonide). Has a synergistic effect on the inhibition of root resorption. Both eliminates pulp space infectin as well as suppresses inflammation
- *Calcitonin:* It is a polypeptide hormone. Resorbing cells are the only cells that have receptors for calcitonin. Use has been proposed in an attempt to control the resorption process. It directly inhibits osteoclastic activity, both *in vivo* and *in vitro* by suppressing the motility of osteoclasts thereby suppressing the inflammation.
- *Bisphoshonates,* commonly used drug in this category is *Alendronate.*
- Amino acids,Taurine is used for the purpose of suppressing the inflammatory root resorption.

EXTERNAL REPLACEMENT RESORPTION

When extensive damage occurs to the innermost layer of the periodontal ligament, competitive healing events take place. Healing from the socket wall and healing from adjacent periodontal ligament occurs, simultaneously.[39] The development of replacement resorption depends on both the degree of damage to the periodontium at the time of injury, and the extent to which the viability of the periodontal ligament cells remaining on the root surface are maintained. If less than 20% of the root surface is involved, a transient ankylosis may occur, which can later be resorbed due to functional stimuli, provided the tooth in the healing period is stabilised with a splint which allows a minimum amount of mobility, or is non-splinted. In larger injuries, a permanent ankylosis is created.

The tooth thus becomes an integral part of the bone remodelling system, the resorbing cells being, primarily, osteoclasts. Subsequently, osteoblasts replace the resorbed areas of the root with bone.[43] In children, replacement resorption leads to loss of ankylosed teeth usually within 1-5 years. In adults, replacement resorption occurs more slowly, often allowing the tooth to function for many years.

Diagnosis:

Clinically, the affected tooth is immobile, and exhibits a high percussive tone. Radiographically, the periodontal ligament space is absent, and a direct union is seen between alveolar bone and the root. In time, infra-occlusion relative to adjacent teeth can be seen both clinically and radiographically.[12]

Treatment:

While appropriate endodontic therapy is effective in the treatment of external inflammatory resorption, replacement resorption cannot be arrested or repaired.

CHAPTER 6: CLINICAL VARIANTS OF ROOT RESORPTION

Fuss et al. in 2003 proposed a clinical classification of root resorption based and the stimulating factors affecting root resorption. According to them the etiology of root resorption requires two phases: injury and stimulation. Injury is related to non-mineralized tissues covering the external surface of the root, the precementum, or internal surface of the root canal, the predentin. The injury is similar to several types of root resorption and may be mechanical following dental trauma, surgical procedures, and excessive pressure of an impacted tooth or tumor. It may also occur, following chemical irritation, during bleaching procedures using hydrogen peroxide 30% or other irritating agents. Denuded mineralized tissue is colonized by multinucleated cells, which initiate the resorption process.[16]

However, without further stimulation of the resorption cells, the process will end spontaneously. Repair with cementum-like tissue will occur within 2-3 weeks if the damaged surface does not cover a large surface area. If the damaged root surface is large, bone cells will be able to attach to the root before the cementum-producing cells; ankylosis is the result of this process. Continuation of the active resorption process is dependent on a common stimulation factor of the osteoclastic cells, either infection or pressure. Its origin is different for each type of root resorption. Therefore, the various types of root resorption should be identified according to the stimulation factors. When these stimulating factors are identified, it will be possible to reverse the process by removing the etiological factor.[18]

PULPAL INFECTION ROOT RESORPTION

The most common stimulation factor for root resorption is pulpal infection. Following injury to the precementum or predentin, infected dentinal tubules may stimulate inflammatory process with osteoclastic activity in the periradicular tissues or in pulpal tissues, consequently initiating external or internal root resorption. Clinically, teeth are usually not symptomatic in the early period of the process, and resorption may be seen at this stage only in radiographs. However, as the process progresses, the teeth may become symptomatic and periradicular abscesses may develop with increasing tooth mobility. Radiographically, radiolucency is observed in the external root surface of the dentin and adjacent bone, or in the internal root canal dentinal walls.

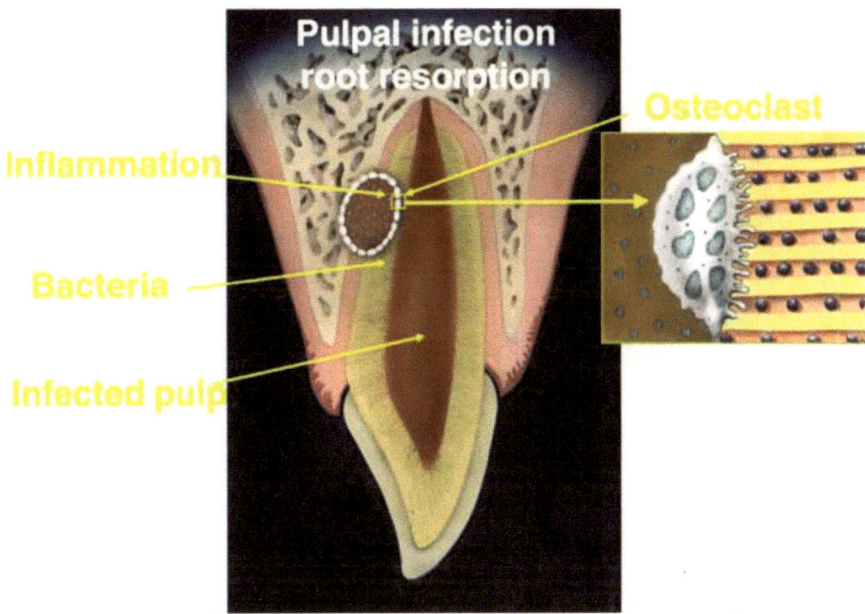

(Courtesy Dr.Zvi Fuss)

Treatment

The resorbing cells in internal resorption are pulpal in origin. Hence, pulpectomy will remove the granulation tissue and blood supply of these cells. For this reason, a pulpectomy alone is a predictable treatment form in this type of resorption. For external resorption, it is critical to control the pulpal bacteria that act as a stimulant for the resorptive process. Bacterial stimulation removed from the dentinal tubules can predictably arrest this type of root resorption. Calcium hydroxide for 6-24 months is the intracanal medicament of choice for treatment of external pulpal infection. Its strong antibacterial effect and low solubility create a long-term effect in the root canal, and remove the stimulation factor from the main canal. Calcium hydroxide also increases the pH of dentin (8.0-10.0), and therefore inhibits the activity of osteoclastic acid hydrolases in the periodontal tissues and activates alkaline phosphatases. However, the pH of the medium surrounding roots containing calcium hydroxide for 10 days with patent dentinal tubules does not change significantly.

The low solubility of calcium hydroxide and buffering effect in dentinal tubules do not allow permeability of hydroxyl ions through dentinal tubules. The antibacterial effect of calcium hydroxide with no additives in the dentinal tubules is significantly weaker than electrophoretically activated calium hydroxide or calcium hydroxide with additives, such as IKI or copper. The new intracanal medicament, Activ Point (Activ point, Roeko, Langenau, Germany), which contains chlorhexidine 5%, has shown significantly stronger antibacterial effect in dentinal tubules to a depth of 500 mm compared to calcium hydroxide or irrigation with chlorhexidine alone.[5]

PERIODONTAL INFECTION ROOT RESORPTION

Bacteria from the periodontal sulcus may penetrate patent dentinal tubules, coronal to the epithelial attachment, and exit apical to the epithelial attachment without penetrating the pulpal space. Consequently, the damaged area of the root surface is colonized by hard tissue resorbing cells, which penetrate into dentin through a small denuded area, causing the resorption inside the root to spread.[25] At the first stage, the resorptive process does not penetrate the pulp space because of the protective layer of predentin, but rather spreads around the root in an irregular fashion. With time, the process may penetrate into the root canal. Additionally, periodontal infection resorption will include the alveolar bone adjacent to the resorption lacuna in the tooth.

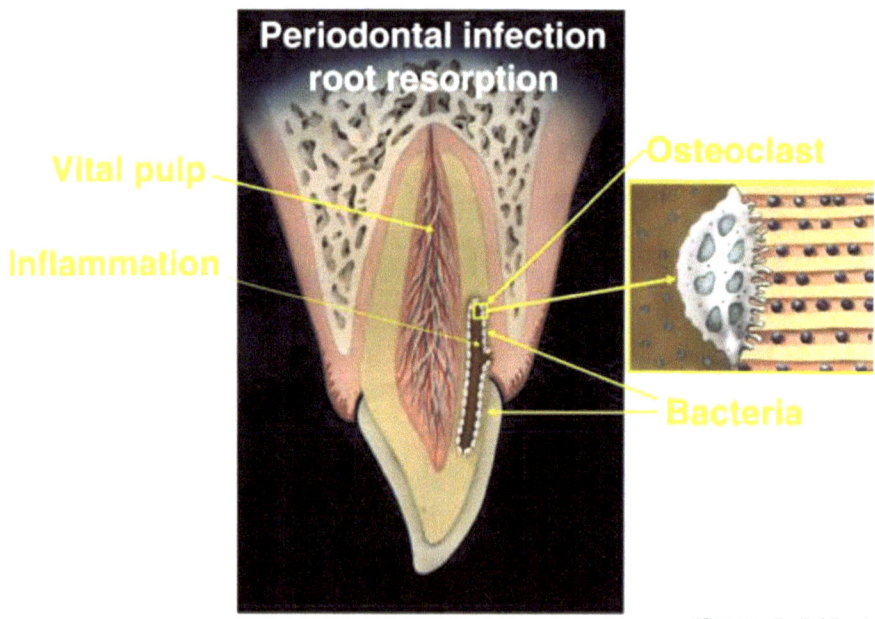

(Courtesy Dr.Zvi Fuss)

Radiographically, periodontal infection resorption can be seen as a single resorption lacuna in the dentin usually at the crestal bone level, expanding to the coronal and apical direction. With progression of the process, radiolucency may be observed at the alveolar bone adjacent to the resorption lacuna of the dentin.[27]

Treatment

As predictable and long-term disinfection of the periodontal sulcus is not possible, the most effective therapy is to expose the resorption lacuna orthodontically or surgically, and to remove the granulation tissue. The resorptive defect should be shaped as a cavity with retentive areas and restored with composite resins or amalgam according to esthetic demands. Endodontic treatment is necessary only when there is perforation to the root canal. Where perforation is strongly suspected or ascertained, root canal treatment may be performed prior to the surgical exposure of the resorption lacuna. If the resorption lacuna is with minute external entrance openings, it can be cleaned out and obturated from the root canal instead of adopting a surgical approach. Follow-up examinations are especially important to determine that the resorptive process has been arrested.[30]

ORTHODONTIC PRESSURE ROOT RESORPTION

One complication of orthodontic treatment is the apical root resorption, with injury originating from the pressure applied to the roots during tooth movement. Continuous pressure stimulates the resorbing cells in the apical third of the roots, a possibility of significant shortening of the root. Teeth are asymptomatic and the pulp is usually vital unless the pressure of the operative procedure is high, which disturbs the apical blood supply. Radiographically, orthodontic pressure resorption is located in the apical third of the root, and no signs of radiolucency can be observed in the bone or the root.

Treatment

Removal of the source of the pressure results in cessation of the resorption, therefore no root canal treatment or operative procedure is needed.[45]

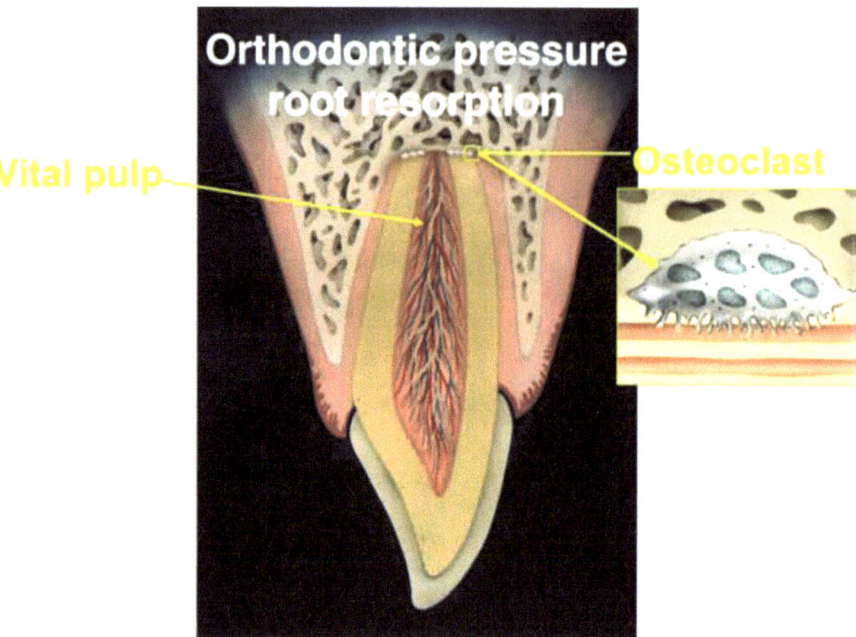

(Courtesy Dr.Zvi Fuss)

IMPACTED TOOTH OR TUMOR PRESSURE ROOT RESORPTION

Pressure root resorption can be observed during eruption of permanent dentition, especially of maxillary canines (affecting lateral incisors) and mandibular third molars (affecting mandibular second molars). Tumors and osteosclerosis impinging on the root of the tooth could also be an etiological factor for pressure resorption. Tumors that produce root resorption are most frequently those in which growth and expansion are not rapid, such as cysts, ameloblastomas, giant cell tumors, and fibrosseous lesions. This type of root resorption is asymptomatic with vital pulp throughout the process unless the impacted tooth or tumor is located near the apical foramen, disturbing the blood supply to the pulp.[36] Radiographically, the resorption area is located adjacent to the stimulation factor, the impacted tooth,or the tumor.There are no radiolucent areas as no infection is involved in the process. The site is filled with the stimulation factor, the impacted tooth,or the tumor.

Treatment

As the stimulation factor is related to bodily objects in the bone, surgery is necessary to remove the pressure and arrest the process. In this case, prognosis is no good.

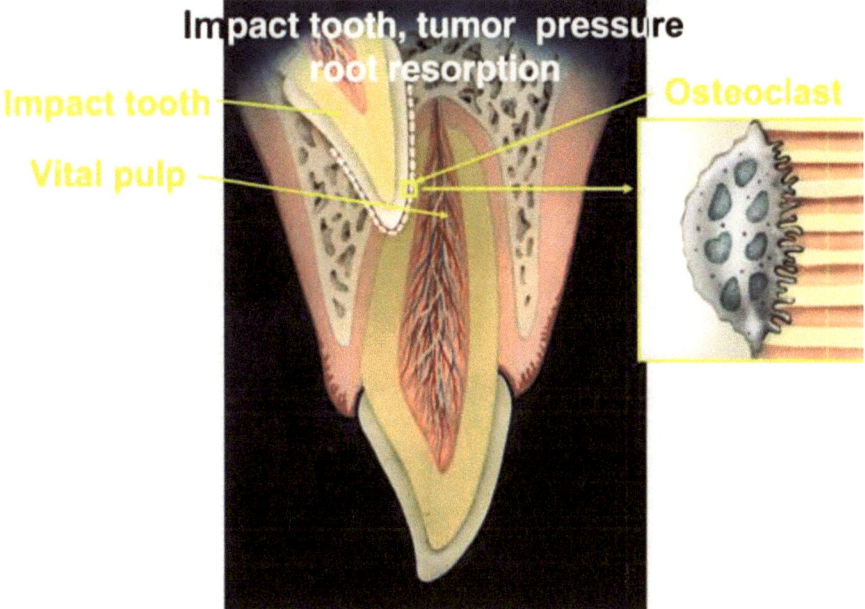

(Courtesy Dr.Zvi Fuss)

ANKYLOTIC ROOT RESORPTION

In severe traumatic injuries, injury to the root surface may be so large that healing with cementum is not possible, and the bone may come into contact with root surface without an intermediate attachment apparatus. This phenomenon is termed as '*dentoalveolar ankylosis*'. Normally the bone is resorbed and formed physiologically in a remodeling process without any specific stimulation with organic tissues protecting dentin. Osteoclasts are in direct contact with the mineralized dentin in the exposed root surface after severe trauma to the root surface. Therefore, resorption can occur without any further stimulation and the bone is laid down instead of the dentin. The process may be reversed if less than 20% of the root surface is involved. Clinically, ankylotic teeth lack the physiological mobility of normal teeth. This is one diagnostic sign for ankylotic resorption. In addition, these teethusually have a special metallic percussion sound and if the process continues, they are in infra-occlusion. Radiographically, resorption lacunae are filled with bone, and the periodontal ligament space is missing. No radiolucent areas are observed, and at some stage, the whole root may be replaced by bone.[55]

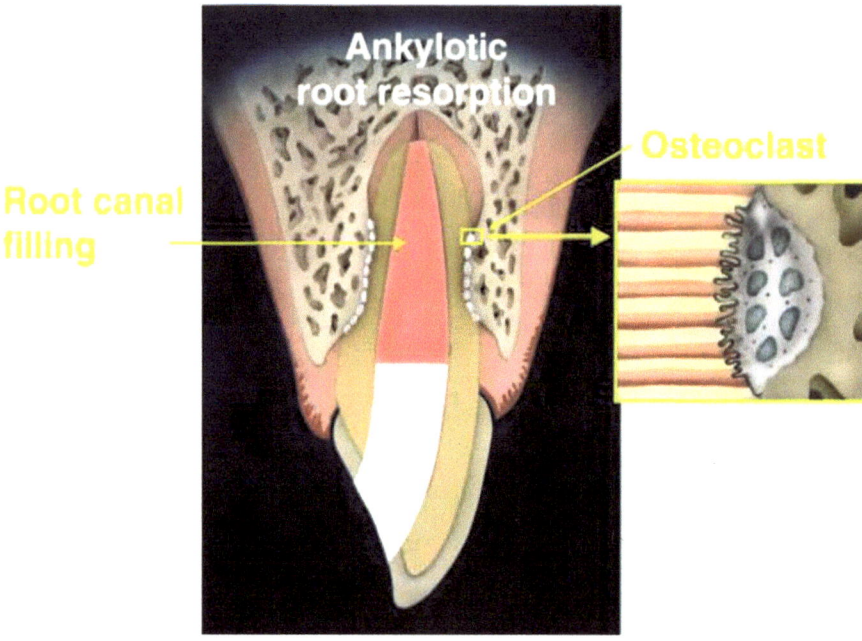

(Courtesy Dr.Zvi Fuss)

Treatment

As there is no stimulation to remove, there is no predictable treatment available at present. The rate of tooth resorption varies and cannot be controlled by the patient or by the operator. Prevention by minimizing periodontal ligament damage immediately following an injury is the only treatment. The best approach is immediate replantation or placing the tooth in milk or other suitable solution to prevent dehydration of the periodontal cells. Functional splint is recommended for placement for 7-10 days, and root canal treatment to prevent pulpal infection root resorption .[41]

CHAPTER 7: TRANSIENT APICAL BREAKDOWN

It is a temporary phenomenon in which the apex of the tooth displays the radiographic appearance of resorption which is invariably followed by surface resorption and / or obliteration of pulp canal. Injured periradicular tissue generally returns to normal following repair 1 year after trauma.[62]

The breakdown process is related to: the type of injury and the stage of root development

Etiology

- ❖ Moderate injuries to the pulp
    - ➢ Subluxation
    - ➢ Extrusion
    - ➢ Lateral luxation
- ❖ Moderate combined injury to the peridontal ligament and the pulp in mature teeth
- ❖ Other causes
    - ➢ Infections
    - ➢ Orthodontic treatment
    - ➢ Occlusal insult to the periodontium

Radiographic evaluation

There will be transient localised change in the size of the apical periodontal ligament space with blunting of the apex from surface resorption. Pulp canal obliteration may be occasionally seen.

Treatment

As the condition is usually asymptomatic no treatment is indicated.

CHAPTER 8: RESORPTION DUE TO SYSTEMIC CAUSES

Even with systemic diseases that cause bone resorption, roots of teeth show remarkable resistance; unless associated with the following condition:[19]

- ❖ Hormonal disturbances such as *renal dystrophy* in which there is an increased oxalate concentration in blood with associated precipitation in hard tissues which causes resorption.
- ❖ Genetic factors
  Resorption of no apparent cause seen in members of the same family
- ❖ Systemic diseases and endocrine disturbances
  - ➢ Hypoparathyroidism
  - ➢ Calcinosis
  - ➢ Gaucher's syndrome
  - ➢ Hyperparathyroidism
  - ➢ Turner's syndrome
  - ➢ Paget's disease (osteitis deformans)
  - ➢ Herpes zoster
  - ➢ Following radiation therapy

Features: Resorption in systemic disturbances usually occurs at the apex of teeth. Any teeth can be affected. Morse in 1974 found that the resorption process is usually present bilaterally.

Treatment : Treatment of underlying systemic disease may cause resorption to cease.

CHAPTER 9: IDIOPATHIC ROOT RESORPTION

Idiopathic external root resorption is a rarely reported condition which has been observed in single or multiple teeth. Pathological root resorption is related to several local and systemic factors. By definition, if an etiological factor cannot be identified for root resorption, the term "idiopathic" is applied. Two types of idiopathic root resorption have been observed; namely, apical and cervical. Cervical root resorption starts in the cervical area of the teeth and progresses toward the pulp. In the apical type the resorption starts apically and progresses coronally causing a gradual shortening and rounding of the remaining root.[21]

Patients with idiopathic root resorption are commonly asymptomatic clinically with an occasional complaint of tooth mobility, so the condition is usually found in routine radiographic examination. According to literature review of Cholia et al, the idiopathic apical root resorptions were slightly more common in the upper jaw and molar region than in the lower jaw and single root teeth; however, these differences were not statistically significant. Resorption also were more frequent in males aged between 14-39 years. Minimal apical external root resorption may be present in all permanent teeth and has been attributed to a variety of causes. However, up to now only numerated cases of idiopathic apical root resorption have been reported in the literature.

CONCLUSION

Early detection is essential for successful management and outcome of root resorption. Root resorption have several local and systemic predisposing factors. Hence, patients with a history of one or more predisposing factors should be monitored closely for initial signs of root resorption.Cone beam computed tomography appears to be a promising diagnostic tool for confirming the presence, appreciating the true nature, and managing the internal and external root resorptions. In addition to the 2-D slices, 3-D reconstruction enables further assessment of the area of interest which enables the right treatment modality for the real pathology. When correctly diagnosed, the treatment of root resorption is relatively simple, with good or even excellent prognosis. However, in cases where the resorption has perforated the root, the tooth structure may have become too weak, and elimination of infection can also be more difficult. However, with proper treatment and use of modern endodontic techniques and materials, the prognosis of even perforated cases is fairly good.

REFERENCES

1. Senem Y.O. Diagnosis and Treatment Modalities of Internal and External Cervical Root Resorptions: Review of the Literature with Case Reports. Int Dent Res 2011;1:32-37

2. Haapasalo.M , Endal.U. Internal inflammatory root resorption: the unknown resorption of the tooth. Endod Topics 2006; 14: 60–79.

3. Yip.L, Fiona H.M and Sandler P.J. Two Cases of Molar Root Resorption. Dent Update 2003; 30: 200-204.

4. Jacobovitz .M , Lima R.K. Treatment of inflammatory internal root resorption with mineral trioxide aggregate: a case report. Int Endod J 2008; 41:905–912.

5. Patel. S, Ricucci. D, Durak. C, Tay. F. Internal Root Resorption: A Review. J Endod 2010; 36:1107–1121.

6. Martin Trope, Noah Chivian ; Root Resorption : Pathways of Pulp Cohen and Burns, 6th Edition.

7. Leif.K Tronstad.Principles of endodontic practice.3rd edn

8. Rugh.P, Brudvik.P. Root resorption beneath the main hyalinized bone. Eur J Orthod. 1994;16(4):249-63

9. Laux M, Abbott PV, Pajarola G, Nair PN. Apical inflammatory root resorption: a correlative radiographic and histological assessment. Int Endod J. 2000 Nov;33(6):483-93

10. Consolaro.A. The concept of root resorptions or Root resorptions are not multifactorial, complex, controversial or polemical. Dental Press J Orthod 2011;16(4):19-24.

11. Geoffrey S., Heitherray. Invasive cervical resorption : An analysis of potential predisposing factors. Quintessence Int. 1999:30:83-95.

12. Andersen M, Lund A, Andreasen JO, Andreasen FM. In vitro solubility of human pulp tissue in calcium hydroxide and sodium hypochlorite. Endod. Dent. Traumatol 1992;8:104-108.

13. Patel.S , Kanagasingam.S. External Cervical Resorption: A Review. J Endod 2009;35:616–625

14. Chan E.K.M , Darendeliler M.A. Exploring the third dimension in root resorption. Orthod Craniofacial Res 2004;7: 64–70

15. Finucane. D, Kinirons M.J. External inflammatory and replacement resorption of luxated, and avulsed replanted permanent incisors: a review and case presentation. Dent Traumatol 2003;19:170-174.

16. Wedenberg .C , Zetterqvist .L. Internal Resorption in Human Teeth- A Histological, Scanning Electron Microscopic, and Enzyme Histochemical Study. J Endod 1987;13(6):255-259.

17. Khojastepour.L, Bronoosh.P, Azar.M. Multiple Idiopathic Apical Root Resorption: a Case Report. J Dent 2010; 7(3):165-169.

18. Nunes .E, Silveira F.F, Soares J.A, Marco A. H. Treatment of perforating internal root resorption with MTA: a case report. J Oral Sci 2012; 54(1): 127-131.

19. Fuss Z, Tsesis I, Lin S. Root resorption – diagnosis, classification and treatment choices based on stimulation factors. Dent Traumatol 2003:19:175-182.

20. M. Laux, P.V. Abbott, G. Pajarola and P.N.R. Nair. Apical inflammatory root resorption : a correlative radiographic and histological assessment. Int Endod J 2000;33:483-493.

21. Ne RP, Witherspoon DE, Glutman JL: Tooth resorption. Quint Int.1999;30:9-25.

22. J.O. Andreasen : Response of oral tissues to trauma. Text Book and Color Atlas of Traumatic injuries to the teeth, 3rd edn, Copenhagen and St. Louis : Munksgaard and C V Mosby, 1994

23. Text Book and Color Atlas of Traumatic injuries to the teeth, 3rd edn, Copenhagen and St. Louis : Munksgaard and C V Mosby, 1994

24. Noah Chivian, Root resorption. Pathways of Pulp Cohen 5th edition

25. Text Book and Color Atlas of Traumatic injuries to the teeth, 3rd edn, Copenhagen and St. Louis : Munksgaard and C V Mosby, 1994

26. Martin Trope : Root resorption due to dental trauma. Endodontic Topics : 79:2002.

27. Cabrini R, Maisto O, Manfredi E. Internal resorption of dentin: histopathologic control of eight cases after pulp amputation and capping with calcium hydroxide. Oral Surg Oral Med Oral Pathol 1957;10:90–96.

28. Yango Pohl, Andreas Filippi, Horst Kirschner. Results after replantation of avulsed permanent teeth. I. Endodontic considerations. Dent. Traumatol 2005; 21:80-92.

29. E. Cotti, D. Lusso and C. Dettori : Management of apical inflammatory root resorption : report of a case. International Endodontic Journal (1998) 31, 301-304.

30. Mauleg LA, Wilcox LR, Johnson W. Examination of external apical root resorption with scanning electron microscopy. Oral Surg 82:83-93, 1996.

31. Vier FV, Figuliredo JAP, : Prevalence of different periapical lesions associated with human teeth and their correlation with the presence of extension of apical external root resorption. International Endodontic Journal, 35, 710-719, 2002.

32. Vier fv, Figueiredo JAP. Internal apical resorption and its correlation with the type of apical lesion. Inter Endod J 2004;37:730-737.

33. R.S. Nance, D. Tyndall, L. G. Levin, M. trope. Diagnosis of external root resorption using TACT (Tuned – aperture computed tomography) Endod Dent. Traumatol 2000;16:24-28.

34. Mente J, Seidel J, Buchalla W, Koch MJ. Electronic determination of root canal length in primary teeth with and without root resorption. International Endodontic Journal, 35, 447-452, 2002.

35. Fuss Z, Mizrahi A, Lin S, Cherniak O, Weiss EL : A laboratory study of the effect of calcium hydroxide mixed with iodine or electrophoretically activated copper on bacterial viability in dentinal tubules. International Endodontic Journal 35, 522-526,2002.

36. Igor Tsesis, Shaul Lin, Ervin I. Weiss, Zvi Fuss. Dentinal pH changes following electrophoretically activated calcium hydroxide ions in the root canal space of bovine teeth. Dent. Traumatol 2005. 21:146-149.

37. Shaul Lin, Ofer Zukerman, Ervin I. Weiss, Yardena Mazor and Zvi Fuss, : Antibacterial efficacy of a new chlorhexidine slow release device to disinfect dentinal tubules. Journal of Endodontics, Vol. 29, No.6, June 2003.

38. Lui JN, Sae-Lim V, Song KP, Chen NN. In vitro antimicrobial effect of chlorhexidine – impregnated gutta percha points on enterococcus faccalis. International Endodontic Journal 37, 105-113,2004.

39. Kee-yeon kum, Joo-Hyun Park, Yun-Jung Yoo, Bong-Kyu Choi, Hyun-Jung Lee, Seung Jong Lee. The inhibitory effect of Alendronate and Taurine on osteoclast differentiation mediated by Porphyromonas gingivalias sonicates in vitro. Journal of Endodontics, Vol. 29, No.1, 28-30; 2003.

40. Levin L, Bryson EC, Caplan D, Trope M.: Effect of topical alendronate on root resorption of dried replanted dog teeth. Dent Traumatol 2001; 17:120-126.

41. Bryson EC, Levin L, Branchs F, Abbott PV, Trope M : Effect of immediate intra canal placement of ledermix paste on healing of replanted dog teeth after extended dry times – Dent traumatol 2002;18:316-321.

42. Wong KS, Sae-Lim V. The effect of intra canal ledermix on root resorption of delayed – replanted monkey teeth. Dent. Traumatol 2002;18:309-315.

43. Iqbal MK, Bamaas NS. Effect of enamel matrix derivative (EMDOGAIN) upon periodontal healing after replantation of permanent incisors in Beagle dogs. Dent.Traumatol 2001; 17:36-45.

44. Filippi A, Pohl Y, Von Arx T. :Treatment of replacement resorption with emdogain preliminary results after 10 months. Dent traumatol 2001; 17:310.

45. Barrett EJ, Kenny DJ. Avulsed permanent teeth : a review of the literature and treatment guidelines. Endod. Dent. Traumatol 1997; 13: 153-163.

46. Iwaya S, Ikawa M, Kubota M. Revascularization of an immature permanent tooth with apical periodontitis and sinus tract. Dent. Traumatol 2001:17:185-187.

47. Vanderas AP, Effects of intra canal medicaments on inflammatory resorption or occurrence of ankylosis in mature traumatized teeth ; a review. Endod. Dent. Traumatol 1993; 9:175-184.

48. Trope M, Moshonov J, Nissan R, Buxt P, Yesilsoy C. Short VS : Long term calcium hydroxide treatment of established inflammatory root resorption in replanted dog teeth. Endod Dent Traumatol 1995;11:124-128.

49. Selma Cristina Cury Camargo, Giulio Gavini, Carlos Eduardo Aun, Douglas waterfield, Jeffery M. Coil. Diffusion of calcitonin through the wall of the root canal. (Journal to be found.

50. Geoffrey S. Heithersay. Clinical, radiographic and histopathologic features of invasive cervical resorption. Quintessence Int. 1999, 30:27-37.

51. K. Patel, U.r. Darbar and K. Gulabivala – External cervical resorption associated with localized gingival overgrowth. International endodontic Journal 35, 395-402,2002.

52. P. Carrotee. : Calcium hydroxide, root resorption, endo-perio lesions. British Dental Journal, Vol. 197, No. 12, Dec. 25, 2004.

53. Euiseong kim, Kee – Dcog Kim, Byoung – Duck ROL, Yong Sikcho, Seury – Jong Lee. Computed tomography as a diagnostic aid for extra canal invasive resorption. Journal of endodontics, vol. 29, 463-465, 2003.

54. Geoffrey S. Heithersay : Treatment of invasive cervical resorption : An analysis of results using topical application of trichloracetic acid, curettage, and restoration. Quintessence Int. 1999;30:96-110.

55. Lee GP, Lee MY, Lum SoY, Poh RSC, Lin K.C. Extra radicular diffusion of hydrogen peroxide and pH changes associated with intra coronal bleaching of discolored teeth using different bleaching agents. International Endodontic Journal, 37:500-506,2004.

56. Loomba K, Govila C.P., Loomba A. Internal resorption –Review and case report. (Endodontology –

57. Cecilia Wedenberg, and Lars Zettergvist. Internal resorption in Human teeth – A histological scanning electron microscopy, and enzyme histochemical study. Journal of endodontis, Vol. 13, No.6, June 1987.

58. K. Gulabivala and L. J. Searson: Clinical diagnosis of internal resorption : an exception to the rule. International Endodontic Journal (1995)28:255-260.

59. B. Thilander, P. Rygh, K. Reitan. : Tissue reactions in Orthodontics. Orthodontics – current principles and techniques, 3rd edition, Graber, Vanarsdall.

60. Bender I.B, Margaret R. Byers, Katsuci Mori, Periapical replacement resorption of permanent, vital, endodontically treated incisors after orthodontic movement : Report of two cases. Journal of Endodontics Vol. 23, No.12, Dec. 1997.

61. Paula A. Villa, Giovanni Oberti, Cesar A. Moncada, Olga Vasseur, Alejandro Jaramillo, Diego Tobon, and Jaime A. Agudelo: Pulp – dentine complex changes and root resorption during intrusive Orthodontic tooth movement in patients prescribed Nabumetone. J Endod 2005;31:45-51.

62. 81st General Session of the International Association for Dental Research (June 25-28, 2003) 0169 Healing of Orthodontically Induced Root Resorption by Ultrasound in Man T. El-Bialy, I. El-shamy

63. W. Schulte and D. Lukas : The Periotest Method. International Dental Journal (1992) 42, 433-440.

64. Andresen M, Mackie I, Worthington H.: The periotest in traumatology . Part I. Does it have the properties necessary for use as a clinical device and can the measurements be interpreted " Dent. Traumatol 2003;19: 214-217.

65. Mackie I, Ghrebi S, Worthington H. Measurement of tooth mobility in children using the periotest. Endod dent traumatol 1996, 12;120-123.

66. Lee S-I, Jung I-Y, Lee C-Y, Choi SY, Kum K-Y. Clinical application of computer aided rapid prototyping for tooth transplantation. Dent. Traumatol 2001;17:114-119.

67. Boyd KS. :Transient apical breakdown following subluxation injury : a case report. Endod. Dent. Traumatol 1995; 11:37-40.

ABOUT THE AUTHOR

Dr. Vineet R.V is currently a faculty member at Sree Mookambika Institute of Dental Sciences, India. He received his Bachelor of Dental Surgery degree from the reputed Tamil Nadu Dr.MGR Medical University and obtained his Master of Dental Surgery degree from the prestigious Rajiv Gandhi University of Health Sciences with high academic excellence.

The author has many research publications in several national and international indexed journals to his credit, and has also authored books related to the field of dentistry. He has been included in the editorial review board of various peer reviewed national and international scientific journals. Furthermore, he has presented scientific papers at various national and international conferences. His research field includes endodontic microbiology, retreatment endodontics, laser endodontics, regenerative endodontics, and dental composites.